Teamwork in Palliative Care

To John

with love from

Vicki

Jun 1990

Teamwork in Palliative Care

A multidisciplinary approach to the care of patients with advanced cancer

ROBIN HULL, FRCGP
Macmillan Senior Lecturer in Palliative Care
Department of General Practice, Birmingham University Medical School

MARY ELLIS MSc, SRN, RCNT, RNT CertEd(Fe)
Director of Education
St Mary's Hospice, Birmingham

VICKI SARGENT RGN, RCNT, CertEd(Fe)
Tutor
St Mary's Hospice, Birmingham

RADCLIFFE MEDICAL PRESS
OXFORD

© 1989 Radcliffe Medical Press Ltd
15 Kings Meadow, Ferry Hinksey Road, Oxford OX2 0DP

British Library Cataloguing in Publication Data

Hull, Robin, 1931 –
Teamwork in palliative care.
1. Terminally ill patients. Care
I. Title   II. Ellis, Mary   III. Sargent, Vicki
362.1′75

ISBN 1 870905 26 1

Printed and bound in Great Britain
Typeset by Advance Typesetting, Oxfordshire

Contents

Foreword

It is always encouraging when professionals of different disciplines work together. It is especially so when their co-operation results in a publication such as 'Teamwork in Palliative Care'.

The concept of hospice care has spread rapidly in the last twenty years and now covers most of the English speaking world. (A beginning is being made to get it into Europe.) However, education in this work, now known as Palliative Medicine, has not kept pace with all the goodwill efforts being made. One is often conscious of a lack of understanding of what is the true philosophy that inspires this, and what is really involved in this care.

This book should go a long way in helping to remedy this lack, and I congratulate the authors on their far-sightedness and expertise in producing it.

MONICA PEARCE M.B.E., S.R.N., S.C.M.(Hon), M.Soc.Sc.
Chairman, Council of Management
St. Mary's Hospice, Birmingham

Preface

In the past teaching of palliative care to medical students at Birmingham Medical School had been restricted to a few lectures and a brief visit to a hospice. In 1989 the general practice attachment in the final year was expanded from three to four weeks, thus providing an opportunity to increase palliative care teaching and its formal assessment.

This book began as a series of notes for this new course. It soon became apparent however that the handout for the new course was a book in itself. Since multidisciplinary groups were increasingly being taught at St Mary's Hospice it was logical to expand the book to include nurses, social workers and others as well as medical students. The first drafts were therefore discarded and the present book emerged as a team approach to the problems of looking after a patient with preterminal and terminal disease.

Fundamental to an understanding of advanced cancer are the simple concepts of epidemiology, pathology and preventive and curative care. The first chapters in this book address these points before examining the two major tasks of palliative care, namely, communication with the patient, his relatives and other carers; and symptom control. These salient features of palliative care are dealt with at length in chapters five to eight. However, symptoms are not just physical so separate chapters are devoted to psychological and spiritual problems. Where cure is no longer possible the help that patients receive from less orthodox methods of care become important; and a section therefore examines the methods of complementary care.

The new epidemic of AIDS poses special problems for palliative medicine which are discussed at length. Later chapters look at the stress that may arise among those who care for patients with advanced cancer and how education can help everyone involved. Care continues after the death of the patient and special attention must be paid to the bereaved and this point is emphasized in the book.

These tasks have been drawn together to show how the team may function to ensure optimum care of patients. The epilogue looks to a future where the principal role of the hospice will be to teach better standards of care for all who bear the strain of any chronic disease. Appendices list useful information about drugs, helping agencies and the question of euthanasia.

This book is for those who care. It is hoped that they will consider their work and see how different contributions can add up to a greater whole.

DR ROBIN HULL
Macmillan Senior Lecturer in Palliative Care
Department of General Practice
Birmingham University Medical School

1 Introduction

This book is written for new entrants to general practice, junior hospital staff and nurses involved in the care of people with advanced cancer at home or in hospital. Some may question the validity of a book aimed at such different readerships. This is because there is a traditional and stereotyped view of the relative roles of doctors and nurses in the provision of care. Traditionally, the medical profession is seen as the more 'important'; doctors take decisions and nurses carry them out. Perhaps because of the increasing professionalism of nurses, with a stronger academic base of research, the traditional view of the doctor—nurse relationship is changing and there have been increasing tendencies for nurses to assume far greater responsibility for patient care than before. The growth in popularity and acceptance of the transatlantic concept of the nurse practitioner[1] is a good example of this change. At the same time there has been a change in the structure of medicine from one predominantly masculine to an increasingly feminine profession; men are moving into nursing where the 10% of nurses who are men hold half of the most important jobs. This change in role of the two professions is most marked in palliative medicine.

When a person is very ill with widespread metastatic cancer, the first need is for expert nursing care, with attention to bowel function, pressure areas and empathetic appreciation of the hundred little symptoms and the many, and often major, physical, emotional, spiritual and social problems of severe illness. The second need is for an understanding doctor, skilled in communication and in symptom control. Palliative care reaches its very best when the different skills of the two professionals are combined. Teamwork is essential, whether care is undertaken in the patient's home, in hospital or in a hospice. Sometimes it may be necessary for the doctor to lead the team, quite as often it will be the nurse who should do so. The trick of good interdisciplinary care depends on mutual respect for each other's different skills, experience and knowledge so that such alteration in leadership is easy and unthreatening to both professionals.

This is why a doctor, experienced in general practice, and two nurses with wide general experience who have come to co-operate in the field of palliative care make no apology for addressing this book to students and new practitioners of both professions in and out of hospital. It is only by starting to learn together that the required mutual respect can be established early and interprofessional threats be diminished.

This does not alter the fact that it is difficult to get the mix of such a book right. Inevitably because of differing backgrounds there may be quite a marked variance in the knowledge base of students and qualified members of both professions. So it will be that some of the information in this book may seem too simple, but simplicity is rarely a fault and it is often useful to reiterate basic principles. Again, we make no apology for sometimes telling some of our readers things they already know. There is a lovely remark attributed to Mark Twain which is apt in this context:

'It ain't what I don't know as makes me a fool,
but what I do know as ain't so.'

Cancer is a complex concept: it consists of many distinct diseases of widely differing seriousness and symptomatology. It is also surrounded by a dense cloud of mythology, folk belief and superstition.

A 33-year-old patient, dying in hospice with melanomatosis remarked to a group of visiting students 'The fear of cancer is worse than cancer'. This remark should be remembered by all who look after cancer patients because it underlines the importance of good communication to allay the patient's terror. Such terror is often based upon ignorance about this group of diseases. The best antidote is understanding, and that can only come through frank and open discussion with informed carers.

The task of cancer care can be summed up as:

'To cure sometimes
To relieve often
To comfort always.'

The relief of fear and the comfort which that brings is always within the reach of the combined skills of a caring team of health and other workers (Table 1.1).

Table 1.1   Possible members of the caring team.

Hospital	Community	Others
Dietician		
Gynaecologists	Ambulance driver	
Haematologists	Community physician	Bank managers
Hospital chaplain	Dietician	Friends
Nurses	District nurses	Lovers
Occupational therapists	General practitioners	Ministers of religion
Oncologists	Health visitors	Neighbours
Otorhinolaryngologists	Home care nurses	Pets
Orthopaedic surgeons	Home help	Relatives
Pathologists	Macmillan nurses	Solicitors
Physicians	Marie Curie nurses	Undertakers
Physiotherapists	Occupational therapists	
Porters	Practice nurses	
Radiographers	Receptionists	
Radiologists	Social workers	
Radiotherapists	Speech therapists	
Social workers	Stoma care nurses	
Speech therapists		
Stoma care nurses		
Students		
Surgeons		
Ward cleaners		

Attitudes

For a while one of us (RH) was invited to work with the Professor of Oncology at the Free University of Amsterdam. One day in outpatients he was examining a young man whom it was hoped was cured of his seminoma. While admiring the patient's prosthesis the doctor asked the patient what part his general practitioner had played in the management of his illness. Astonishingly the pleasant young Dutchman became extremely angry and said: 'Until I got cancer my doctor was a close personal friend, afterwards he did not want to know.' How do you react to such an anecdote? Do you feel the young Dutchman was right to be so angry? From time to time throughout this book we will return to this story to explore the attitudes of patient and doctor.

There is other evidence of the reduction in community care for the very ill; in 1900, 70% of patients died at home but by 1984 this proportion was reduced to 30%.

Consider this statement:

'Cancer is a common, fatal, painful, undignified disease
and in consequence greatly to be feared.'

Is cancer common?

That depends on what is meant by common and the standpoint. In hospices almost everyone has cancer; in hospital wards many may have it; but the general practitioner with a list of some 2000 patients sees only six or seven new cancers a year (Table 1.2).[2]

Table 1.2 Numbers and types of cancer patients consulting annually in a practice of 2000.

Cancer site	No. of persons
All cancers (new 7)	15
Lung	2
Breast	2
Gut	1
Stomach	1 in 3 years
Cervix	1 in 5 years
Brain	1 in 10 years
Thyroid	1 in 20 years

Certainly cancer is a common cause of death with one in three people dying of cancer in western Europe. But one only dies once and the expectation of life is 70−75 years so this even occurs only every 200−250 man years; does this make it common?

Is cancer always fatal?

Increasingly, malignant disease is curable. Enormous advances have been made and cancers of childhood, Hodgkin's disease and seminoma, for example, now carry a far better prognosis with the result that the life-shortening effect of cancer has been greatly reduced. The cancers of later life are less amenable to treatment and, with the increasing age of the population, are becoming more common. Even in the sixth and seventh decades cancer can often be controlled or slowed to permit greater expectation of life and this has had the effect of increasing multiple primary cancer. Patients with two or more primary tumours are not infrequent.

Is cancer always painful?

Cancer in its early stages is painless—therefore making diagnosis more difficult. Cancer produces pain through tissue destruction, trauma, pressure, nerve involvement, ischaemia or secondary infection. About 70% of advanced cancers give rise to pain; 30% seldom, if ever, do. With modern techniques of analgesia, pain should very seldom be a major or prolonged problem.

Is cancer undignified?

It can be especially when causing visible destruction in the head and neck. It also may cause loss of mobility, change in physical appearance, and bowel or urinary incontinence. But so may many other chronic diseases. Loss of dignity and autonomy are often more attitudinal than real, and skilled care may minimise them or at least render them no more important in cancer than in other diseases.

Management

The management of cancer in hospital or in the community is complex. It depends more upon the identification of the patient's and carer's attitudes, preconceptions, knowledge and fears about this hugely disparate group of diseases than upon the complexities of oncological management. Management of cancer depends on knowledge about the disease and its treatment, but it also demands highly developed skill in communication and the correct approach or attitude. Teaching usually focuses on the inculcation of knowledge. Though there will be much fact in this book, this will often be regarded as less important than the improvement in the reader's communication skills and the challenging of his or her attitudes.

Palliation is a branch of cancer care and is as important as prevention, diagnosis, management and terminal care, all of which are different from palliative care. Palliative care is defined as 'that care provided for patients in whom, after exact diagnosis, attempts to cure have been considered and abandoned'.

It follows that the aim of palliative care is the maximization of the patient's physical, emotional, social and spiritual quality of life. Terminal care, sometimes spoken of synonymously with palliative care, concerns the management of death itself and, though it may be part of palliative care, is distinct from it. Palliative care may be required for years, even decades, while terminal care is agonal, lasting only hours or days.

In the following chapters the subject of epidemiology and pathology of cancer will be reviewed briefly and in a chapter on prevention and curative care the division of labour between primary, secondary and tertiary care, is examined with particular reference to the hiatus in care which may arise when a patient is passed from one level of care to another. The complaint of the Dutchman with the seminoma is discussed again in this context. This leads to the subejct of communication between the patient and his or her carers. Detailed chapters deal with the control of physical and other symptoms. Because many patients seek alternative care for relief of their disease and its symptoms considerable space is given to a review of some forms of complementary medicine. The role of such alternative therapy is discussed with possible explanations for the success that some patients report of it.

Later chapters look at the special problems of AIDS and aspects of interdisciplinary teaching and learning for all who care for patients with advanced cancer both in and out of hospices. Finally, one of the appendices lists drugs in order to present the reader with details of names, dosage and indications for the drugs mentioned in the text.

References

1   Stilwell, B., Greenfield, S., Drury, V.W.M. & Hull, F.M. (1987) A nurse practitioner in general practice: working style and pattern of consultations. *Journal of the Royal College of General Practitioners* **37**: 154–157.
2   Fry, J. (1988) *GP Data Book*. MTP Press, Lancaster.

Further reading

Souhami, R. & Tobias, J. (1987) *Cancer and its Management*. Blackwell Scientific Publications, Oxford.
Hancock, B.W. & Bradshaw, J.D. (1986) *Lecture Notes on Clinical Oncology*, 2nd edn. Blackwell Scientific Publications, Oxford.

2 Epidemiology of cancer

The word epidemiology derives from Greek: *epi*, among; *demos*, the people; and *logos*, science or study, hence the 'study of what is among the people'. Alternatively, it is said to be about 'taloia' fever (There's A Lot Of It About). Epidemiology is the study of how a disease, in this case cancer, behaves in populations. Populations may consist of those who live in a given town or country or they may be selected by other distinctive criteria such as age, sex, social class and so on. The study of disease in populations teaches about causes and, perhaps, how they may be prevented. The fact that cancers of different kinds may be more common in some groups of individuals than in others may indicate ways in which those specific groups can be helped, perhaps in their life styles or in their attitudes. Even in epidemiology we find that the way towards lessening some of the effects of cancer may be through the alteration of attitudes.

We have already looked at the 'commonness' of cancer, which depends on the measurement of incidence or prevalence:

Incidence = *New cases* occurring in a standard population at a given time

Prevalence = *All cases* present in a standard population at a given time

The overall incidence of all cancers is slowly increasing (though there may be large fluctuations in the incidence of individual cancers). This is because the disease becomes much more common with increasing age and, with the demographic shift in numbers of the aged, so incidence increases.

The prevalence is increased because of greater expectation of life following correct diagnosis and treatment of cancer. This is particularly true of primary brain tumours where incidence is generally low but which, because of increased life expectancy, now make up some 10−15% of all cancer cases in local hospices.

Causation of cancer

Epidemiology helps to reveal causes of cancer by linking disease to factors which may influence it. The trouble is that observed association between two occurrences does not mean they are causally linked. An example of this is provided by the observation that ice-cream sales rise at a time when deaths from drowning are most common. At first sight one might think that ice-cream caused drowning, but the association is with a third variable: hot weather which encourages swimming and increases the sales of ice-cream. Thus, when there is an association between observed events this does not necessarily indicate a causal relationship.

When trying to understand what causes an individual cell to become cancerous it is easiest to start with the control of cell replication. Cells consist of cytoplasm and a nucleus which contains the genetic material. Deoxyribonucleic acid (DNA) is the basis of the genetic code which acts as the blueprint controlling cellular growth and reproduction. DNA is a long chain consisting of an intertwined double helix of polynucleotides. Polynucleotides are chains of nucleotides and nucleotides are complex organic compounds consisting of a sugar molecule plus a phosphate molecule plus a nitrogenous base. These bases are adenine (A), cytosine (C), guanine (G) and thymine (T).

The genetic code is a combination of A C G T (like the dash and dot of Morse code) which might be represented schematically as

C A G A C T G A C T A G

Mutation may occur when, for a variety of reasons, this code is upset, for example:

C A G A T T G A C T A G

Such mutation is usually lethal to the cell and so mistakes are self-destructive; some produce changes which are beneficial to the species but some programme the cell to undergo malignant change.

DNA, like life itself, is both very fragile and at the same time very durable, however it is susceptible to damage by a number of physical, chemical or biological factors. Changes in DNA structure probably occur commonly; many are self-destructed, many more are destroyed by the immune system which recognizes the cell with a new genetic structure as 'non-self' and kills it.

Thus cancer may be caused by mutant change *and* by failure of the immune system to destroy the abberant cells.

Many factors are related to the cause of cancer, either by encouraging mutation or by preventing the destruction of the resulting abnormal cells. These causative factors may be inherited (from nature) or acquired (from nurture).

Inherited factors (nature)

Familial predispositon

Some childhood cancers are inherited because of familial predisposition; for example some retinoblastomas are inherited as a dominant trait. Neuro- and nephroblastomas may also have a familial element.

Chromosomal abnormalities

Some chromosomal abnormalities are associated with increased cancer, for example, acute leukaemia in Down's syndrome (trisomy 21), or breast cancer in Klinefelter's syndrome (XXY).

Immunodeficiency syndromes

There are rare inherited syndromes associated with immunodeficiency (such as Wiskott−Aldrich syndrome in which various malignant tumours are common). There are also some inherited syndromes which appear to be premalignant and which are associated with an increased risk of cancer, for example, polyposis coli and bowel cancer or xeroderma pigmentosum and skin cancer.

Histocompatibility antigens

Some cancers may be associated with the histocompatibility antigens, human leucocyte antigens (HLA). These particular antigens are important in tissue typing in order to check compatibility of donor transplant tissue. The antigens are genetically determined and play an important part in determining susceptibility to disease. Some inherited variations of these antigens appear to be related to cancer and may partly explain clustering of malignancy in certain families.

Environmental factors (nurture)

Irradiation

Radiation is a naturally occurring phenomenon; visible light makes up a very small proportion in the middle of the range of natural radiation. At one end of the scale there are the radio wavelengths (which are the longest) and at the opposite end are the very short X-rays and γ-rays. The longer the wavelength of these radiations, the less the energy, so when one reaches the very short wavelengths of X- and γ-rays there is much more energy. Therefore, radiation from sunlight which contains infra-red, visible light and ultraviolet radiation may be an important cause of skin cancers. X-rays may also cause skin cancer, as many of the early radiologists discovered to their cost. Some radioactive ores have caused lung cancers among miners, people working with luminous watch dials have developed bone cancer, and many of those subjected to the atomic bomb explosions of Nagasaki and Hiroshima have since developed thyroid cancer.

Chemicals

A number of inorganic compounds may be carcinogenic, for example: asbestos may cause lung cancer, particularly mesothelioma; arsenic is important in the causation of skin and lung cancers; chromium is also associated with lung cancer; and nickel with tumours of the lung and nasal sinuses. Similarly a number of organic chemicals such as benzine derivatives may play a part in the causation of cancers of the lung, skin and bladder. PVC (polyvinyl chloride) is implicated in cancer of the liver. Many such cancer-causing organic substances are present in cigarette smoke. The presence of nitrites in foodstuffs is also suspected of carcinogenesis; nitrites are converted to nitrous acid in the stomach and may react with amines in food to form nitrosamines with the potential, as yet unproven, of carcinogenesis.

Some moulds which may occur in stored food produce substances called aflatoxins, which are thought to be a cause of cancer of the liver. Primary liver cancer is rare in the western world, but is very common in Mozambique where it is thought that the presence of the aflatoxins is due to moulds affecting stored peanuts. It is likely that aflatoxin acts by enhancing other cancer-producing factors such as the hepatitis B virus. The association between tobacco-smoking and lung cancer is now accepted, but the position of alcohol is unclear though it appears to be associated with several cancers, such as cancer of the oesophagus, oral cavity and maxillary antrum, but whether it is causative (or like ice-cream and drowning!) is uncertain.

A number of drugs used by doctors may play a part in the cause of cancer but will probably require decades before their carcinogenic dangers are fully appreciated, just as the early radiologists had to wait many years to discover that their exposure to X-rays and γ-rays had induced malignancy. Of drugs in current use which might be expected to have a potentially carcinogenic effect, the cytotoxic and immunosuppressive drugs seem most likely. Some tumours, such as those of the breast and prostate, are hormone-responsive and it is thought that hormone imbalance may contribute to their causation. Other tumours may result from therapeutic use of hormones, for example in treatment of menopausal symptoms.

Viruses

The association between virus infection and tumours has been known since Rous, working at the Rockefeller Institute in 1911, discovered that a sarcoma of chickens could be transmitted by a virus. However, the exact relationship between viruses and cancer is not clear. Burkitt's lymphoma is caused by the Epstein–Barr virus which also causes infectious mononucleosis. It appears that malarial infection modifies the immune response of some individuals, altering the host's relationship with the virus which is then able to stimulate malignant change. Other examples include hepatitis B virus and hepatoma, and human immunodeficiency virus (HIV) and Kaposi's sarcoma. Herpes simplex virus 2 and human papilloma virus may play a role in the causation of cancer of the cervix, although the precise relationship is not clearly understood.

Immunological factors

Once potentially malignant change occurs, most cells are destroyed by the immune system. Immune deficiency may occur for many reasons, it may be associated with treatment as, for example, the immunosuppression induced to prevent rejection after tissue transplants, with infections such as AIDS (acquired immune deficiency syndrome); and also with many malignancies. In certain cases of stress there is depression of lymphocytic activity. This may account for the increased incidence of certain infections, such as infective mononucleosis, at times of examination stress or the increase in infection and cancer following bereavement (see Chapter 15, p. 123).

Chronic irritation

This is one of the oldest known associations with cancer, for example, pipe-smoking and cancer of the lip.

Geographical factors

Some cancers are more common in particular parts of the world (Table 2.1). Such observation could be explained in terms of nature or nurture. The higher incidence of breast cancer in America than in Japan might be due to some inherited predisposition in American women or to some environmental factor which increases the risk of this particular growth. Alternatively, protective factors in either nature or nurture in Japan may reduce breast cancer there.

Table 2.1 Regional incidence of specific cancers.

Site	High incidence	Low incidence
Lung	Western world	Japan
Breast	USA	Japan
Stomach	Japan	South & West Africa
Uterus and cervix	India	Israel
Bladder	Egypt	
Postnasal space	China	
Liver	Africa, South-East Asia	

The relative importance of nature and nurture influences can be seen more clearly through studying immigrants and their patterns of disease. When people migrate they tend to approximate to the pattern of disease in the host country. Japanese women living in America have a higher incidence of breast cancer, though not as high as native Americans, suggesting that the effect of nurture is stronger than that of nature.

Distribution of specific cancers

The overall prevalence of cancer by age, sex, social class and the site of the primary cancer is shown for regions of England and Wales in Figs. 2.1 to 2.5. (see pages 12–20)

Lung

Cancer of the lung is by far the most common malignancy in the western world. Deaths in England and Wales have risen from 7000 to 35 000 since World War II. It has an overall incidence of 112 per 100 000 males and 27 per 100 000 females in Britain; the incidence is increasing at a rate of 8% in males and 50% in females per decade; it is decreasing in doctors and increasing in nurses. This is almost entirely related to smoking habits. Lung cancer is rare below the age of 25, high in the 60s in men and in the 70s in women. The incidence is highest in the lowest social classes, possibly related to smoking and, in consequence, is high in those areas of Britain of predominantly low social class (see Fig. 2.1a,b,c, pages 12–13).

Breast

The breast is the most common site of cancer in women, and breast cancer is the most common single cause of female death in the age group 40 to 44. It is rare below 30 but rises sharply with age thereafter. There is a familial tendency and the most important single factor is the hormone status of the tumour. Many breast cancers carry cellular receptors or oestrogens and other steroid hormones. In postmenopausal women about two-thirds of breast cancers are oestrogen-receptive, but only a third of cancers are in younger women. Where the presence of a hormone receptor can be established it is possible to predict that the disease will respond to hormone therapy or to oöphorectomy. Formerly, other means of modifying hormonal influences on breast cancer by hypophysectomy and adrenalectomy were sometimes used; the latter has largely been superseded by medical adrenalectomy with aminoglutethimide. Breast cancer is more common in higher social classes and in the presence of fibroadenosis, but is less common with parity and prolonged breast-feeding. These factors probably account for its higher incidence in south and east Britain (see Fig. 2.2a,b,c, pages 14, 15).

Figure 2.1a Deaths from lung cancer (including trachea and bronchus) per 100 000 population by age, sex and standard region 1970 – 72.

Standard region		0 – 14	15 – 44	45 – 54	55 – 64	65 – 74	75 and over	SMR (15 – 64)
England and Wales	M	0.0	4.6	79.8	284.3	585.5	588.4	100
	F	0.0	1.8	24.0	52.8	76.1	80.0	100
North	M	–	6.2	101.5	318.2	591.8	544.8	116
	F	0.1	3.1	34.2	55.7	65.5	66.0	121
Yorkshire and Humberside	M	–	5.5	90.7	295.3	584.6	564.0	107
	F	–	1.9	25.0	50.0	63.0	71.5	98
North West	M	–	6.7	100.3	328.0	643.6	596.5	119
	F	–	2.3	29.6	55.5	73.2	73.3	112
East Midlands	M	–	4.5	68.0	254.4	549.0	498.7	89
	F	–	1.4	18.3	46.9	69.7	63.2	84
West Midlands	M	–	5.0	90.9	295.0	570.7	494.4	106
	F	–	1.6	25.0	45.8	67.1	61.5	92
East Anglia	M	–	4.2	64.4	233.4	506.1	523.3	82
	F	–	0.8	21.9	45.2	62.3	71.2	85
South East	M	0.0	3.5	70.9	282.3	627.6	700.0	96
	F	–	1.7	22.8	60.0	94.9	103.5	107
South West	M	–	2.9	59.9	234.4	478.4	454.3	80
	F	–	1.0	19.1	46.9	69.4	60.7	84
Wales I	M	–	4.6	66.8	249.1	484.2	473.6	87
	F	–	2.0	17.0	36.1	43.1	55.8	72
Wales II	M	–	4.9	70.6	248.9	480.8	478.7	88
	F	–	1.7	16.4	30.6	46.9	39.3	63

Figure 2.1b Incidence of lung cancer (including trachea and bronchus) for metropolitan counties, intermediate and rural aggregates 1974.
SRR = Standardized Registration Rate

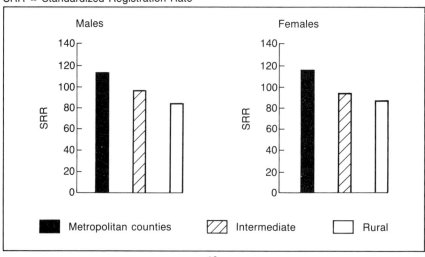

Figure 2.1c Mortality caused by lung cancer (including trachea and bronchus) by sex and standard region 1970 – 72.
SMR = Standardized Mortality Rate

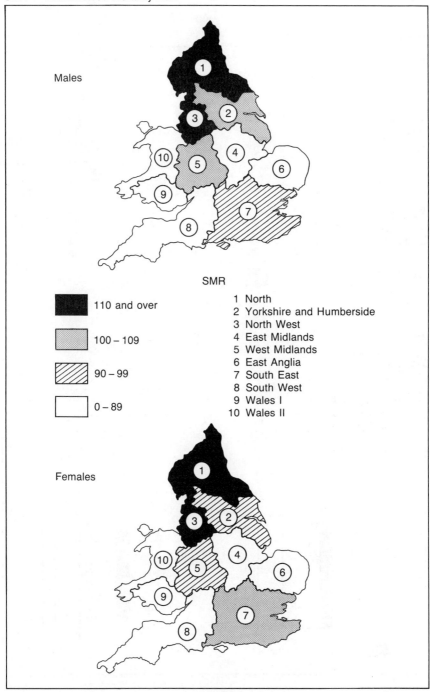

Males

SMR

110 and over

100 – 109

90 – 99

0 – 89

1 North
2 Yorkshire and Humberside
3 North West
4 East Midlands
5 West Midlands
6 East Anglia
7 South East
8 South West
9 Wales I
10 Wales II

Females

13

Figure 2.2a Deaths from breast cancer per 100 000 population by age, sex and standard region 1970 – 72.

Standard region		0 – 14	15 – 44	45 – 54	55 – 64	65 – 74	75 and over	SMR* (15 – 64)
England and Wales	M	–	0.0	0.1	0.7	1.5	3.7	100
	F	–	8.9	61.7	94.2	114.5	166.7	100
North	M	–	–	–	0.9	2.3	6.3	140
	F	–	9.7	58.5	72.4	93.7	138.6	88
Yorkshire and	M	–	–	0.2	0.6	1.7	3.3	100
Humberside	F	–	8.8	61.6	81.8	98.9	141.9	93
North West	M	–	0.0	–	0.4	1.4	4.3	90
	F	–	8.7	56.7	90.5	107.1	153.0	95
East Midlands	M	–	0.0	0.3	1.1	1.4	1.3	100
	F	–	9.2	62.9	103.6	129.7	178.6	106
West Midlands	M	–	0.0	–	0.7	2.1	3.2	104
	F	–	9.7	61.3	97.7	114.6	180.8	103
East Anglia	M	–	–	–	0.4	0.5	2.2	69
	F	–	7.4	53.4	95.7	111.5	165.1	94
South East	M	–	0.0	0.0	0.8	1.7	4.0	109
	F	–	9.0	64.9	101.3	124.0	177.0	106
South West	M	–	0.0	0.2	0.6	0.8	2.8	76
	F	–	6.6	60.8	94.3	118.5	164.3	96
Wales I	M	–	–	0.5	0.6	0.5	4.7	98
	F	–	8.9	60.8	86.2	109.2	158.1	95
Wales II	M	–	–	–	1.5	–	2.2	68
	F	–	9.8	67.1	91.1	92.4	199.6	102

* Male SMR is for all ages

Figure 2.2b Incidence of breast cancer for metropolitan counties, intermediate and rural aggregates 1974.

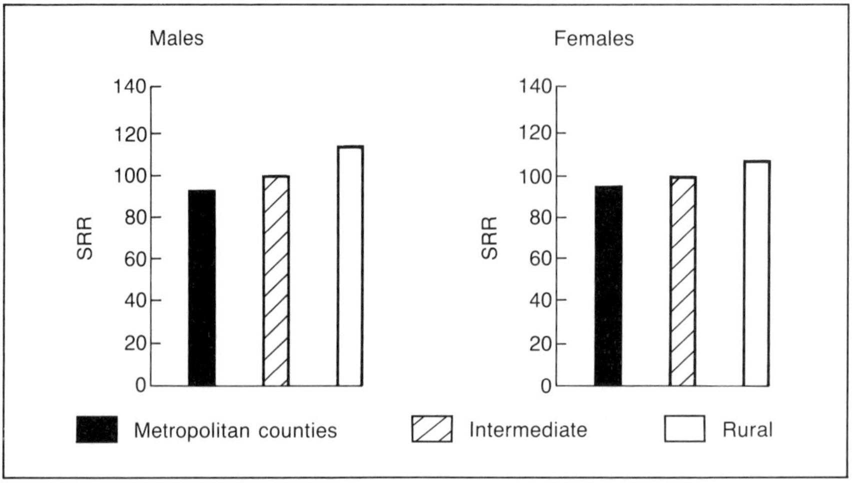

Figure 2.2c Mortality caused by breast cancer by sex and standard region 1970 – 72.

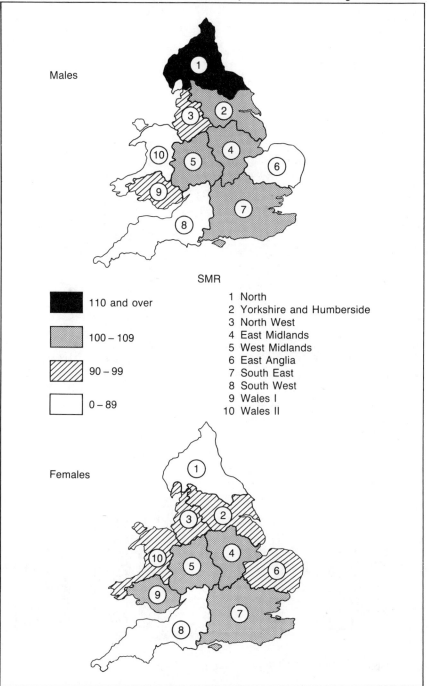

Males

SMR

	110 and over
	100 – 109
	90 – 99
	0 – 89

1 North
2 Yorkshire and Humberside
3 North West
4 East Midlands
5 West Midlands
6 East Anglia
7 South East
8 South West
9 Wales I
10 Wales II

Females

Figure 2.3a Deaths from melanoma and other cancers of the skin per 100 000 population by age, sex and standard region 1970 – 72.

Standard region		0 – 14	15 – 44	45 – 54	55 – 64	65 – 74	75 and over	SMR (15 – 64)
England and Wales	M	0.0	0.8	2.0	3.9	6.9	17.6	100
	F	0.0	0.8	2.8	3.3	4.7	10.6	100
North	M	–	0.7	2.2	3.7	5.1	18.1	100
	F	–	1.2	2.1	2.7	5.4	12.3	96
Yorkshire and Humberside	M	–	0.8	1.6	3.5	6.9	17.2	93
	F	–	0.6	2.4	2.9	4.5	12.1	84
North West	M	0.1	0.4	1.3	4.5	8.0	19.9	84
	F	–	0.8	2.5	2.8	4.1	10.0	89
East Midlands	M	–	0.7	2.5	3.9	5.8	13.9	104
	F	–	0.6	2.7	3.3	4.3	11.0	92
West Midlands	M	0.1	0.8	2.2	4.3	5.7	15.4	106
	F	–	0.8	2.2	2.4	4.7	8.4	80
East Anglia	M	–	0.7	1.0	2.9	9.4	20.7	74
	F	–	0.5	3.4	4.3	3.2	8.7	107
South East	M	–	0.9	2.5	3.8	6.9	16.2	111
	F	0.1	1.0	3.3	3.6	4.8	10.6	114
South West	M	–	0.8	2.3	4.4	6.5	18.2	112
	F	–	0.9	3.3	3.5	5.4	11.4	109
Wales I	M	–	0.8	1.1	2.7	8.0	22.5	76
	F	0.1	0.8	2.6	3.0	6.9	11.8	94
Wales II	M	–	0.5	–	1.5	7.8	33.6	35
	F	–	0.7	0.7	5.6	2.8	10.1	101

Figure 2.3b Incidence of melanoma and other cancers of the skin for metropolitan counties, intermediate and rural aggregates 1974.

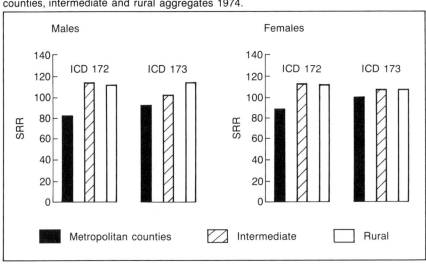

Figure 2.3c Mortality caused by melanoma and other cancers of the skin by sex and standard region 1970 – 72 (ICD 172 and 173).

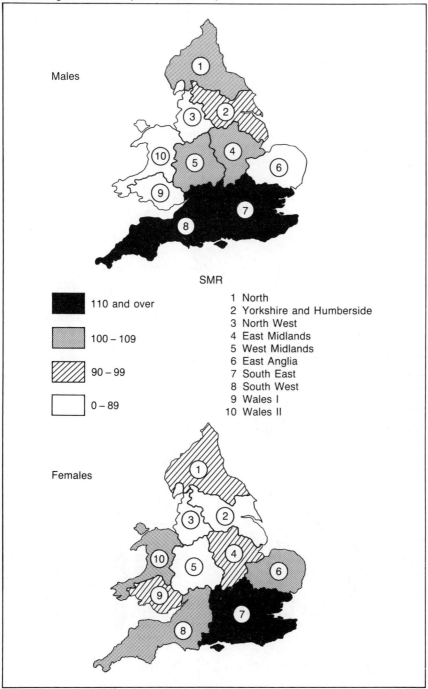

SMR

110 and over

100 – 109

90 – 99

0 – 89

1 North
2 Yorkshire and Humberside
3 North West
4 East Midlands
5 West Midlands
6 East Anglia
7 South East
8 South West
9 Wales I
10 Wales II

Males

Females

Figure 2.4a Deaths from cancer of the stomach per 100 000 population by age, sex and standard region 1970 – 72.

Standard region		0 – 14	15 – 44	45 – 54	55 – 64	65 – 74	75 and over	SMR (15 – 64)
England and Wales	M	0.0	1.5	18.5	68.1	156.7	259.0	100
	F	–	1.0	8.0	25.4	67.0	161.7	100
North	M	–	2.2	19.6	81.4	180.6	295.4	118
	F	–	1.8	10.3	32.3	85.4	203.9	132
Yorkshire and Humberside	M	–	1.4	20.0	65.2	158.0	259.8	98
	F	–	0.9	10.0	28.7	73.7	176.9	113
North West	M	–	1.8	20.4	80.1	180.9	296.3	116
	F	–	1.2	9.9	32.0	81.0	175.5	125
East Midlands	M	–	1.5	18.9	65.3	150.8	253.0	98
	F	–	0.7	9.7	21.5	68.2	161.6	91
West Midlands	M	–	1.3	21.1	76.5	166.4	251.4	111
	F	–	0.9	6.7	27.4	71.9	167.9	100
East Anglia	M	–	1.0	14.0	50.2	137.1	223.0	74
	F	–	0.8	5.7	19.0	49.2	150.6	75
South East	M	–	1.4	17.0	61.1	140.6	242.9	90
	F	–	1.0	6.7	21.3	52.6	142.4	85
South West	M	–	1.6	16.1	57.9	135.6	236.0	86
	F	–	0.7	5.9	19.2	63.6	156.6	75
Wales I	M	0.0	1.6	20.4	83.4	195.4	329.1	119
	F	–	1.4	11.3	34.7	97.9	194.6	137
Wales II	M	–	1.4	19.5	94.2	216.6	302.0	129
	F	–	1.0	6.8	36.2	83.3	197.4	127

Figure 2.4b Incidence of cancer of the stomach for metropolitan counties, intermediate and rural aggregates 1974.

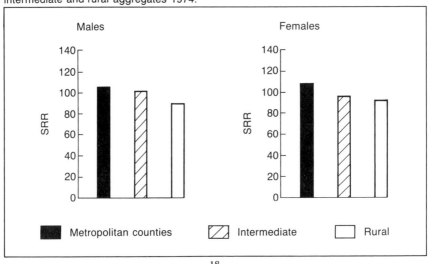

Figure 2.4c Mortality caused by cancer of the stomach by sex and standard region 1970 – 72.

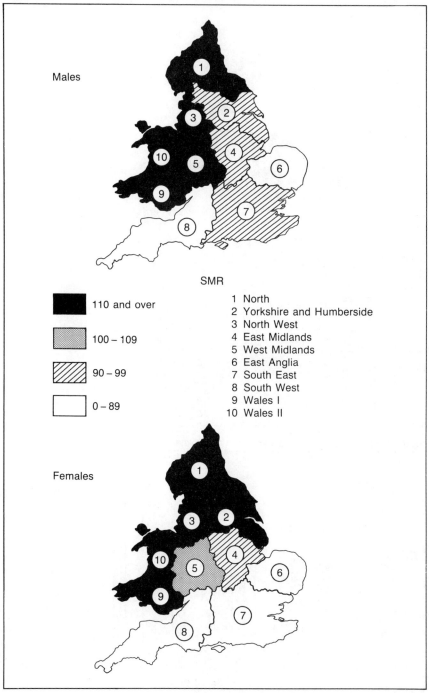

SMR

110 and over

100 – 109

90 – 99

0 – 89

1 North
2 Yorkshire and Humberside
3 North West
4 East Midlands
5 West Midlands
6 East Anglia
7 South East
8 South West
9 Wales I
10 Wales II

Males

Females

Figure 2.5a Mortality from cancer of the cervix uteri by standard region 1970 – 72.

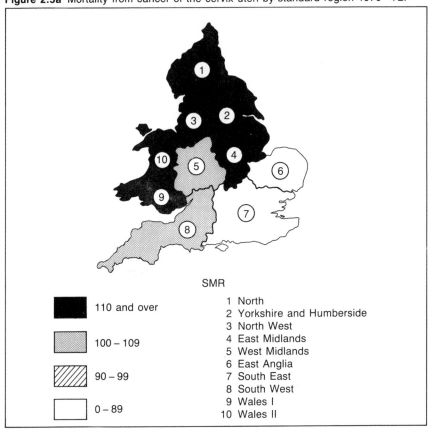

SMR

■ 110 and over

▨ 100 – 109

▨ 90 – 99

□ 0 – 89

1 North
2 Yorkshire and Humberside
3 North West
4 East Midlands
5 West Midlands
6 East Anglia
7 South East
8 South West
9 Wales I
10 Wales II

Figure 2.5b Mortality from cancer of the cervix uteri by social class 1970 – 72.

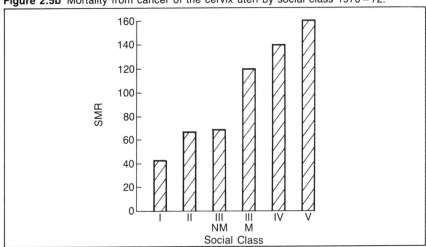

Skin

Skin cancers are common—especially basal cell cancer (rather more than half) and squamous cell carcinoma (a little more than a quarter), with the rest made up of melanomas, lymphomas and other rarer cancers. Skin cancers are more common in fair-skinned people and in parts of the world where there is considerable exposure to sunlight. Thus Australia and South Africa report large numbers of people with skin cancers. In Britain there is an increased incidence along the south coast.

Basal cell carcinoma, or rodent ulcer, is the most common skin cancer (50%). It is more common in men (M:F=5:3) and is most commonly seen above a line drawn from mouth to ear.

Squamous cell carcinomas may occur anywhere in the skin and may also result from sun exposure, possibly influenced by other carcinogenic factors such as arsenic or radiation.

Malignant melanoma is rare, giving rise to less than 2% of all skin cancers, however there has been a considerable rise in its incidence during the 1980s. As with other skin cancers it is related to sun exposure (whether real or from sun-lamps) and is ten times more common in Australasia than in Europe. It is seen most commonly in southern Britain (see Fig. 2.3a,b,c, pages 16, 17) and is almost twice as common in women than men and rare in pigmented skins. It carries a very bad prognosis.

Stomach

Cancer of the stomach was, until recently, one of the most common cancers in western civilization. In parts of Latin America and South-east Asia the incidence is twice that of Britain, and Japanese figures are four times that of Britain. The ratio of male to female is 2:1 and there is a higher incidence in social classes I and II. Gastric cancer usually occurs in the sixth decade and are more frequent in the north and west of Britain (see Fig. 2.4a,b,c, pages 18, 19).

Prostate

This is one of the most common cancers of men and the third largest cause of their deaths from cancer. The incidence of prostatic cancer is difficult to determine since many are found at the removal of 'benign' glands.

Bowel

The bowel is a common site of cancer especially in white races, and is related to diet. It occurs in both sexes and in middle to old age. Small-bowel cancers are rare, accounting for only 5% of all gastrointestinal cancers. Large-bowel tumours, particularly in the sigmoid and rectum, are the second largest cause of cancer deaths in the western world. Large-bowel cancer occurs in the caecum and ascending colon (15%), the recto-sigmoid (40%) and rectum (35%), with three-quarters being visible using sigmoidoscopy.

Gynaecological cancers

Cervix

A great deal is known about the prevention of cancer of the cervix, yet many comparatively young women suffer from this disease. Cervical intraepithelial neoplasia (CIN) is graded according to the severity of cytological abnormality. Carcinoma *in situ* (CIN3) is the most serious. Such a lesion on the cervix may remain quiescent for many years, but as many as 30−40% left untreated will develop into invasive carcinoma. Ninety per cent of cervical cancers are squamous, a further 5% are adenocarcinoma and the remainder a variety of rare lesions.

The disease is extremely rare in nuns and Jewish women. Cancer of the cervix is related to sexual activity, especially the age of commencement and the number of sexual partners. Other factors include high parity, low social class and a history of sexually transmitted diseases, particularly those due to the human papilloma and herpes simplex viruses. There is also an association with smoking but this could either be causal or incidental.

Though this has always been a cancer of younger women, the age of onset of carcinoma of the cervix appears to be falling. Unfortunately attitudes held by society towards consulting about gynaecological symptoms discourage those most in need from screening or reporting symptoms which may indicate genital cancer. Similar attitudes may also have an effect upon consultation for other cancers particularly of the bowel. (see Figs. 2.5a and 2.5b, page 20)

Rarer gynaecological cancers

Endometrial cancer is less common than cervical cancer (ratio of 1:2). It occurs in postmenopausal women and is most common in the nulliparous; it may be associated with obesity and diabetes. Cancers of the ovary comprise about 20% of gynaecological tumours and are of many varieties. They may occur at any age but the incidence increases with age. Vaginal and vulval tumours are rarer cancers which tend to occur in later life.

Uncommon cancers

Brain

Primary brain tumours are rare (about 2% of all human tumours). They occur at all ages, with peak incidences in the first decade and between 50 and 60 years of age, with equal sex incidence, and in white races more than black. Although they are rare their prevalence is increasing due to longer survival.

Kaposi's sarcoma

We are likely to see more of this formerly very rare tumour, which used to be limited to Ashkenazim Jews around the Mediterranean littoral. It occurs as the initial manifestation of AIDS in 30% of cases, especially in white homosexuals (less in blacks and in i.v. drug users). The lesions in Kaposi's sarcoma appear as multicentric pink to purple skin or oral tumours.

Further reading

Hancock, B.W. & Bradshaw, J.D. (1986) *Lecture Notes on Clinical Oncology*, 2nd edn. Blackwell Scientific Publications, Oxford.
Souhami, R. & Tobias, J. (1987) *Cancer and its Management*. Blackwell Scientific Publications, Oxford.

Office of Population Censuses and Surveys Cancer Research Campaign. Cancer Statistics incidence, survival and mortality in England and Wales. HMSO London 1981.

3   Pathology of common tumours

The pathology of tumours is important in palliative care because their local and distant spread may give rise to particular problems in symptom control.

Classification of tumours

The word tumour simply means swelling. *Cancer* is the Latin name for a crab which was thought to represent a corrosive evil. Carcinoma, which really should only be applied to malignant tumours arising from epithelial tissue, is derived from the Greek work *karkinos* which also means a crab. A sarcoma arises from the fleshy structures, muscle and connective tissue, and the name derives from the Greek *sarcoma*, meaning flesh.

Tumours may be either benign or malignant, though the distinction may sometimes be far from clear because benignancy and malignancy represent ends of a spectrum with a large grey area in between. Table 3.1 classifies tumours found in different tissues.

Malignant tumours arising from epithelial cells are the commonest cancers and are called carcinomas. Malignancies arising from connective tissue such as bone, muscle, fibrous or fatty tissue, are sarcomas. Cancers may also arise from blood-forming or lymphatic tissues and are designated lymphomas. Those arising from nerve tissues are neuroblastomas, neurofibrosarcomas or gliomas depending on whether they derive from the nerves themselves or from the glial cells, the supportive tissues of the central nervous system (CNS). Some tumours arise from embryonic tissue or from the testes or ovaries; this group comprises a mixture of tumours of childhood or early adulthood.

Some common cancers

Lung

Lung cancer occurs in several forms of which four account for the vast majority (Table 3.2). Lung cancers metastasize, especially to brain bone and liver, and

Table 3.1 A classification of tumours.

Tissue	Tumour	
	Benign	Malignant
Epithelium		
Squamous	Papilloma	Squamous cell carcinoma
Transitional	Papilloma	Transitional carcinoma
Glandular	Adenoma	Adenocarcinoma
Connective tissue		
Fibrocyte	Fibroma	Fibrosarcoma
Fat cell	Lipoma	Liposarcoma
Muscle (voluntary)	Leiomyoma	Leiomyosarcoma
Muscle (involuntary)	Rhabdomyoma	Rhabdomyosarcoma
Bone	Osteoma	Osteosarcoma
Lining of blood vessels	Haemangioma	Haemangiosarcoma
Cartilage	Chondroma	Chondrosarcoma
Blood-forming and lymphatic tissues		
Red blood cell	Polycythaemia vera	
White blood cell		Leukaemia
Lymphoid cells	Lymphoma	Lymphoma
Plasma cells		Myeloma
Central nervous system		
Neurocytes	Ganglioneuroma	Neuroblastoma
CNS supportive tissue (glial cells)	Gliomas	Gliomas
Nerves	Neurilemoma	Neurilemoma
	Neurofibroma	Neurofibrosarcoma
Meninges	Meningioma	Meningiosarcoma
Embryonic and gonadal tissues		
Testis		Seminoma/teratoma
Ovary		Teratoma
Chorion	Hydatidiform mole	Choriocarcinoma
Kidney		Nephroblastoma
Liver		Hepatoblastoma
Nerve tissue		Neuroblastoma
Retina		Retinoblastoma
Others		
Melanocytes	Moles	Malignant melanoma
Liver		Hepatoma

Table 3.2 Features of the four main types of lung cancer.

Type	Prevalence	Histological features	Origin	Prognosis
Squamous cell carcinoma	35%	Keratinization and/or intercellular bridging	Large bronchi	Poor, but better than the others
Small cell carcinoma	25%	Diffuse growth of small, tightly packed cells with granular nuclei	Proximal large bronchi	Very poor
Adeno-carcinoma	25%	Derived from glandular epithelium with acini, papillae and mucus	Peripheral; may arise from areas of fibrosis; is less related to smoking	Intermediate
Large cell carcinoma	15%	Undifferentiated with wide variety of cellular appearance	Distal bronchi	Intermediate

may give rise to special problems such as superior vena caval obstruction and hypercalcaemia (which occurs especially in small cell carcinoma due to the production of parathormone-like substances).

Breast

Almost all breast cancers arise from the epithelium of the lactiferous ducts, are adenocarcinomas and may vary considerably in their degree of malignancy. Breast cancer may spread locally into the skin of the chest wall (cancer *en cuirasse*) or into axillary, supraclavicular, cervical or internal mammary nodes. Distant metastases may occur in lung, liver, bone (especially the axial skeleton) and brain. Like small cell lung cancer, some breast tumours produce parathormone-like substances and may be associated with hypercalcaemia. Lymphoedema of the arm is another common problem which occurs in about 10% of patients with breast cancer. It is frequent in patients who have undergone radical mastectomy and radiotherapy and is due to impairment of venous and lymphatic drainage from the arm. It may also occur in a leg following destruction of pelvic lymphatic or venous drainage.

Skin

On the whole, basal cell carcinomas, or rodent ulcers, are relatively benign since they rarely metastasize and are of low grade malignancy. However they may persist for many years and can be very destructive locally.

Some squamous cell cancers of skin may be very aggressive, particularly in the head and neck or when arising from mucocutaneous junctions such as the anus or vulva. Squamous cell carcinomas may spread locally to regional nodes (especially when the primary tumour is undifferentiated) and less frequently to distant sites.

Malignant melanomas metastasize to the liver and sometimes to the brain. The usually poor prognosis varies with the degree of aggressiveness of the tumour.

Stomach

Gastric cancer spreads locally to nodes along the lesser curve, to the coeliac nodes and to the porta hepatis. Distant metastases may occur in the lung, liver or by direct transperitoneal spread to the ovary (Krukenberg's tumour).

Prostate

Prostatic cancer metastasizes to bone and often presents with the symptoms of bony pain. Many cancers of the prostate respond to hormone therapy with oestrogens or to orchidectomy.

Bowel

Bowel cancers metastasize via the portal vein to the liver. Less often they may metastasize to lung, brain or bone.

Cervix

In advanced cases direct spread occurs downwards into the vagina and laterally into the parametria and pelvis. Lymphatic spread leads to involvement of nodes along the common iliac vessels and aorta. Blood-borne metastases are relatively rare but may involve lung, liver and bone.

Other gynaecological cancers

Cancers arising from the body of the uterus are usually adenocarcinomas which may spread directly into adjacent pelvic structures. Lymphatic spread occurs in the nodes along the common iliac vessels and aorta but may also involve the inguinal and distant lymph nodes. Blood-borne metastases are unusual, though commoner than with cervical cancer, and may occur in lung and bone.

Ovarian cancers are very varied, some 27 types of tumour have been classified. Local spread occurs throughout the peritoneal cavity leading to omental and diaphragmatic secondaries. Distant metastases may occur in the liver, lung and central nervous system.

Rare tumours of the vagina and vulva spread locally to involve the adjacent perineal or pelvic structures.

Brain

Primary brain tumours are rare, but produce many symptoms associated with raised intracranial pressure, altered brain function, epilepsy, dementia or loss of cranial nerve function. The commonest are gliomas, many of which arise from astrocytes, the main supporting cells of the brain. Secondary tumours commonly arise from lung or breast cancers or from melanoma. Less often brain secondaries may arise from cancers in the ovary, testis, gut, bladder, kidney, pancreas, liver and from lymphomas.

Further reading

Hancock, B.W. & Bradshaw, J.D. (1986) *Lecture Notes on Clinical Oncology.* Blackwell Scientific Publications, Oxford.

Souhami, R. & Tobias, J. (1987) *Cancer and its Management.* Blackwell Scientific Publications, Oxford.

4 Preventive and curative care

The stages of care of cancer patients and the usual division of labour between various carers are summarized in Figure 4.1. This chapter examines those stages before palliative care begins.

Stage	No disease →	Pre-symptomatic phase →	Symptomatic phase →	Debilitating phase →	Dying phase
Treatment	Health education	Screening	Early diagnosis	Early treatment	Later treatment	Palliative care	Terminal care

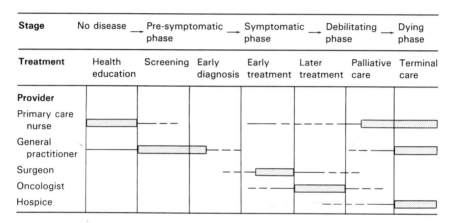

Provider
Primary care nurse
General practitioner
Surgeon
Oncologist
Hospice

Figure 4.1 Stages of care of cancer patients.

Prevention

General practitioners and nurses have a very important role in prevention. Prevention depends on the identification and, where possible, the removal of risk factors. Some genetically determined precancerous conditions such as polyposis coli or xeroderma pigmentosum may require special treatment to lessen the risk of malignant change. For example, there has been a recent case of a 17-year-old daughter of a hospice patient who was dying of cancer of the colon resulting from malignant change in a polypoid colon, who underwent prophylactic hemicolectomy.

More commonly, prevention is directed at the removal of environmental dangers such as industrial chemicals and pollutants of atmosphere, soil or water. Among these, by far the most important is cigarette smoke which has an undoubted association with lung cancer and a probable link with cancers of the stomach, oesophagus, bladder and cervix. The task of weaning people from tobacco is so difficult that it is easy to be nihilistic about it. However, constant counselling by a respected and friendly general practitioner and the primary care team undoubtedly has an effect[1]. Perhaps the most important aspect of such counselling is by example; many doctors have given up smoking, but unfortunately, nurses have been slow to follow suit. The effect of this health education has had greatest effect amongst members of higher social classes; those most at risk are least likely to heed the advice to stop smoking. The single most important factor in campaigns to reduce smoking lies in the respect with which the team is regarded. Members of primary care teams may earn such respect in many ways but one of the most important is in their palliative care of cancer patients. Therefore, the good care of one patient with cancer may help to establish the trust which strengthens the team's ability to prevent disease in others.

Primary care doctors and nurses have great opportunities for health education. This should be a part of every general practitioner's consultation. However, it may still not reach the members of the population most at risk and it is important to make every effort to reach them by seeking opportunities to address audiences (e.g. schools or women's groups). The Women's Institute is a very efficient means of reaching large sections of the community since this nationwide organization has a membership greater than that of all the political parties put together. Women play an enormous part in the health of the nation and therefore comprise an extremely important audience.

Screening populations for early presymptomatic cancer is also important, but certain criteria must be satisfied before screening programmes are undertaken:

1 Is the test to be used sufficiently sensitive?
2 Is the disease curable when detected early?
3 Is the disease common?
4 Are there special populations who should be screened?
5 How frequently is screening necessary?
6 Are there disadvantages in screening?

Several techniques for cancer screening have been suggested and are listed in Table 4.1. Of these only screening for cervical cancer is widely undertaken

Table 4.1 Screening techniques for different cancers.

Disease	Screen
Cervical cancer	Papanicolaous smear
Breast cancer	Self-examination Medical/nurse examination Mammography
Colorectal cancer	Faecal occult blood, routine rectal or sigmoidoscopic examination
Ovarian and uterine cancer	Pelvic examination Pelvic ultrasound
Skin cancer	Self-examination

in Britain since the others do not satisfy the criteria for screening tests. Here, again, there is the problem that those sections of the community who are most at risk are least likely to avail themselves of screening opportunities. Many general practices now have recall systems based on manual or computerized age/sex registers which identify those who need cervical smears. Unfortunately there are still defaulters and these include women at high risk. These women can only be reached by tagging their records and by opportunistic screening when they attend for other reasons. Another inhibiting factor in screening is the fact that a majority of general practitioners are male. Some women find it difficult to talk to male doctors about gynaecological symptoms. Though it may be easier to talk to women doctors it may be easier still to discuss apparently minor genital symptoms with nurses. This delegation of some cervical cytology to nurses is sometimes criticized by doctors because nurses may miss other gynaecological pathology. It is better surely to have some examination rather than none, and nurses can easily report any suspicion of abnormality to the doctor.

Early diagnosis

The early symptoms of cancer may be slight or non-existent, leading to delay in presentation. When they are presented, the symptoms may be non-specific and pose great diagnostic difficulties. Cancer presents to the general practitioner in many ways, from a cryptogenic lesion to one which is all too obvious. In the former, diagnosis may be very difficult leading to delay and multiple investigation or, where the condition is obvious, there may be rapid referral. In both these cases patients may misinterpret the doctor's action—either as incompetence at diagnostic failure or lack of interest because of immediate referral—which can undermine the doctor–patient relationship. This is a common cause of management failure and may give rise to subsequent complaints about the general practitioner's handling of the case. Given that some cancers present with the most trivial and mundane symptoms, it is impossible not to fail on some occasions despite meticulous care. The only safeguard is to maintain a high index of suspicion, to examine frequently and investigate often. All general practitioners will recognize this as an unattainable counsel of perfection which is costly and carries the risk of increased personal somatization.

Though patients should be responsible for their own health they need education for such responsibility. In particular they need to be aware of the seven cardinal symptoms which they should report and which doctors should always take seriously. These are:

1 Any unusual bleeding.
2 Altered bowel habit.
3 Dysphagia.
4 Hoarseness.
5 Unexplained lumps or swellings.
6 Change in appearance of skin lesions such as moles.
7 Unexplained loss of weight.

Unfortunately the majority of cancers are occult and present at a stage when they are already inoperable.

Discussion with the patient

Once suspicion of cancer has arisen in the mind of the carer, early referral will be mandatory except in a few cases of very advanced disease or patient refusal. It will be necessary to give the patient some form of information at this stage and considerable debate always centres on the topic of what this should be. We offer some suggestions of how this might be done, but stress that there is not one correct way. How information is given to patients must vary from case to case as well as varying between carers. However, some principles can be offered.

It is essential that good communication between the patient and carers is established as early as possible. This raises the eternal problem of what, when and how much to tell. If we are honest, often the real reason for not being open with patients about diagnosis is due to our own inadequacy; we do not like giving bad news. However, the thought of enduring the real and imaginary fears associated with cancer treatment by surgery, radio- and chemotherapy without adequate explanation seem far worse than a completely frank, but kindly, statement of diagnosis accompanied by an enthusiastic reassurance that 'this is what we (doctor or nurse and patient) are going to do about it'. It is very important to stress the positive aspects of the individual patient's case so that one never removes hope.

It is important to also remember the words that 'the fear of cancer is worse than cancer' (see p. 2). Counter-arguments in favour of secrecy, however, raise the problem of the patient who wishes to remain in ignorance. It is difficult to believe that, at today's level of general information, people of average intelligence can be unaware of the possibility of cancer, particularly as the disease progresses. Despite this, some people when told the truth will deny within a few minutes that they have ever been told; such denial is a defence mechanism adopted by these individuals and should be respected. In our opinion, however, to not tell a patient the truth and thus to deny access to the help that discussion of his or her fears and worries may bring, is extremely cruel. The common and paternalistic practice of informing the relatives but not the patient must be questioned. This necessarily breaches confidentiality and may give rise to complications if the relatives then forbid the doctor to tell the truth. If, under these circumstances, the relatives insist on secrecy every effort should be made to dissuade them. It is often possible to achieve this by explaining that if everyone is lying to the sick individual, then he or she is cut off from all those who might help with the psychological and spiritual anguish of the disease. Any situation in which a patient is aware that the family or general practitioner is lying cannot do anything but harm relationships.

When the news should be broken is also a thorny question; some argue that it is sensible to wait until there is a definitive diagnosis. It should be borne in mind that the longer the task is left the more difficult it becomes. It is a characteristic of human beings that, when explaining their own symptoms to themselves, the worst possibilities come to mind. Many patients presenting even quite simple symptoms have already thought of some awful explanation for them; for example, a woman presenting with a lump in her breast is nearly certain to have already thought of cancer. It is arguable that the subject might be discussed early in the consultation, even though the lesion may not be cancer at all. If one waits for certainty, which may come at any time from examination to biopsy, the task may have become very much more difficult.

How the news is broken is also problematical and must vary with every individual doctor, patient and circumstance. Certainly it requires time, patience and above all kindness. Such open-ended questions as 'What do you think is the matter?' or 'What do you fear is causing your symptoms?' may lead to the patient using the word cancer, or one of its many euphemisms, first. There is a tremendous advantage gained if the patient introduces the word cancer, as it can then be used openly in conversation. This ventilation of the idea of cancer can be followed with further open-ended questions such as 'What do you understand by cancer?' or 'What does cancer mean to you?' Putting this sort of question is never easy, but will be much more difficult later in the course of the disease. What is more important, is that where there has been such a degree of candour the patient should feel that he or she can trust the doctor and that there is no barrier of falsehood between them.

Referral

Once such a degree of honesty is established, it is possible for the general practitioner to explain why he is referring the patient for further advice and what the consultant may do. He should ensure that the patient will return to discuss the implications of the consultant's advice and to allow further explanation. This seems much more sensible than the earlier paternalistic approach which might, drawn to absurd length, have lead to a doctor saying 'Don't worry it's only a little lump; we'll cut it out, give you some X-rays that may make your skin sore and some pills which may make your hair fall out, but don't worry'.

Referral must be swift, the general practitioner should see that there is minimal delay once suspicion of cancer arises even if this means overriding normal routine and hospital bureaucracy. Referral will usually be by means of a letter, perhaps supporting an earlier telephone call to fix an appointment.

The referral letter should state clearly the history and physical findings of the case, should mention other relevant medical history and medication and, most importantly, should tell the consultant what the patient and, where relevant, what the relatives have been told about the nature of the disease. The letter should also indicate to the consultant that the general practitioner wishes to keep in touch with the patient who should, as a matter of routine, be given a follow-up appointment following the hospital consultation so that the contact is maintained. It is particularly important that the general practitioner sees the patient shortly after the first hospital consultation. Many patients are frightened or overawed by their first hospital visit and may not understand or absorb what they have been told.

Management

The relative roles of carers in the management of a person with cancer may be represented diagramatically (see Fig. 4.1). Unfortunately, a common practice appears to be one of ignoring the cancer patient after referral; for example, the Dutch patient with seminoma (see p. 3). Patients attending outpatients rarely see their own doctors and visits by general practitioners to hospital wards are lamentably few. This is unfortunate though perfectly understandable; general practitioners have plenty to do without seeing to those already under the care of hospital doctors. Ignorance of the complexities of modern oncology may also inhibit their follow-up of patients. But such total handing over to the high technology of a hospital environment is bound to have its effect upon the doctor—patient relationship. Patients may see their doctor as ignorant (many of them come to know more about their chemotherapeutic regimes than their family doctor) or, worse still, uncaring.

Bridging the gap

How can this gap in general practitioner care be bridged? In Birmingham, we are trying out a scheme similar to that of shared obstetric care, in which a co-operation card is held by the patient (see Fig. 16.2, p. 138). It is hoped that this will help to improve communication between the variety of carers looking after an individual. The card will inform the patient not only of the diagnosis but also about his or her progress, as well as explaining symptomatology and side-effects. The card can also be a means of a consultant asking the general practitioner for, say, a full blood count before the next outpatient appointment. Similarly, records can be made by the patient, nurse, general practitioner or anyone else involved. Such a card, by itself, could be counterproductive but used by each carer as a means of exploring whatever physical, psychological, social or spiritual problems the patient is facing can be enormously beneficial. It also has the very important function of bringing the patient together with the appropriate member of the primary care team during the phase of hospital care. This is essential if there is to be continued trust between the patient, his or her family and the team; this is particularly important when the care of the patient moves into the palliative and later terminal phase.

Rehabilitation

Rehabilitation is another important aspect of palliative care. Rehabilitation derives from the Latin *rehabilitare*, to render able again, and means to make fit after disablement or illness, for earning a living or playing a part in the world. The World Health Organization defines rehabilitation as the combined and co-ordinated use of medical, social, educational and vocational measures for training and retraining the individual to the highest possible level of functional ability. As with many WHO definitions this leaves the uncomfortable feeling that all of us, in falling short of goals implied in this definition, are in need of such care. However, it is clear from this definition that rehabilitation needs to begin as soon as the individual is aware of being ill as he or she will immediately develop some reaction to the symptoms. Rehabilitation should commence with the exploration of the patient's fears and anxieties, especially with regard to potential disability and threat to body image.

Specific needs

One of the more common disabilities resulting from treatment is alopecia following radio- or chemotherapy. Wigs of high quality are prescribable by consultants under the National Health Service.

Patients with bowel cancer will often require a colostomy or ileostomy. Some require enormous help in adapting to their new bowel function and altered body image, others find it relatively easy. Patients will also need to learn about potential problems such as stricture, prolapse or soreness surrounding the stoma. Assistance is available from specially trained stoma care nurses and further advice may be obtained from the Colostomy Welfare Group and the Ileostomy Association (see Appendix 2, p. 147, 148).

Special problems may affect patients whose throat cancer has led to laryngectomy. Such patients will need to be taught how to create an oesophageal voice which requires the expertise of speech therapists. Other patients will require prostheses for breast, limb, testicle, or facial deficiencies all of which will require counselling about perceptions of self-image. In addition, there are a great number of aids designed to help mobility, washing, bowel and urinary difficulties and communication. Details of these and of organizations available to provide help and advice are listed in Appendix 2.

References

1 Richmond, R.L., Austin, A., Webster, I.V. (1986) Three year evaluation of a programme by general practitioners to help patients to stop smoking. *British Medical Journal* **292**:803.

Further reading

Doyle, D. (1987) *Domiciliary Terminal Care*. Churchill Livingstone, Edinburgh.

Hancock, B.W. & Bradshaw, J.D. (1986) *Lecture Notes on Clinical Oncology*, 2nd edn. Blackwell Scientific Publications, Oxford.

Souhami, R. & Tobias, J. (1987) *Cancer and its Management*. Blackwell Scientific Publications, Oxford.

Spilling, R. (Ed.) (1986) *Terminal Care at Home*. Oxford University Press, Oxford.

5 Communication in palliative care

Palliative care begins at the point where, after exact diagnosis, attempts to cure have been considered and abandoned. The aim should be the maximization of the patient's quality of life. With such an infinitely variable disease as cancer, palliative care may be required for anything from a few days to several years. Good palliative care depends on two principles: communication and symptom control. Communication is discussed here and the symptom control in chapters 6–10.

Good communication should aim at relieving that fear which is itself worse than cancer. One of the saddest comments made by patients and their relatives is: 'the doctor didn't come, he said there was nothing he could do'. There is always something that one can do by listening and explaining, for the very presence of someone who knows and understands is crucial. That such communication is essential is seen in the frequency with which physical symptoms such as pain, dyspnoea, or nausea become bearable even without drug therapy simply by means of reassurance from a known, trusted and friendly nurse or doctor. In these days of high technology it is not fashionable to stress humanity as an important aspect of the doctor's role, however one has only to ask the very sick for them to confirm that, in their view, this is the physician's most important function. It is not one, however, which can be fulfilled if, like the Dutchman's doctor (see p. 3), trust has already been forfeited.

Good communication depends on listening and talking. The appreciation of verbal and non-verbal hints, suggestions and implications may allow identification of the patient's attitudes, preconceptions and fears. In attempting this, one must be aware of that British characteristic 'the stiff upper lip': the fear of showing emotion. Above all, one needs time for listening, reflecting on half-spoken questions and explanation of fact, tempered with honesty and kindness and discussion in terms the patient can understand. This is not easy, nor are there any hard and fast rules about how it should be done since each situation is unique; doctors and nurses vary in their personalities and skills, patients vary even more and so do each set of circumstances.

Barriers to communication

It is important to be aware of barriers to communication and to try and break them down. Doctors, and probably to a lesser extent nurses, impose many such barriers. Some of these are inherent in the job separating them from patients by gulfs of relative intelligence, culture, class or religion. Barriers begin with the organization of a practice especially with regard to access to the doctor or nurse. The pressures of modern general practitioners are considerable but much can be done to improve access to care. Access depends on many factors such as surgery times, bus timetables and adequacy of public telephones or the absence of car parking or wheelchair ramps.

Receptionists are important because, to an extent, they control the flow of patients and the patient's choice of whether to see a doctor or a nurse. Receptionists often get a bad press and are sometimes referred to as 'the dragons at the gate'. They have a very difficult but essential job which has been well described as helping the team to help the patient. They act as gatekeepers to the practice, trying to assess, as tactfully as possible, the relative urgency of each request for help. To some patients this may seem to be an unwarranted intrusion or even invasion of privacy. In such cases, the receptionist must be prepared to give way; it is, however, essential to rank requests according to urgency in order to avoid chaos. The experienced, tactful receptionist does this routinely, but it is by no means easy. There will always be times when demand exceeds supply of time, energy or patience; nevertheless, care must be taken that such exigencies do not prevent the needy from receiving care which others, less needy but more demanding, may obtain.

Other barriers at the practice reception desk include insufficient staff to answer the many questions which flood in personally or by telephone. There may be physical barriers such as glass partitions or enquiry hatches. There may be a lack of privacy so that the whole waiting room can overhear the conversation between the patient and receptionist. All these factors may deter a patient from making the initial appointment; in many cases of self-limiting disease this will not matter, but it is hard to reconcile such barriers with the often stated exhortation to report symptoms early.

Yet another barrier lies in the aura that surrounds the doctor. It may be hard for doctors themselves to realize that to certain sections of society they represent authority and the establishment and that they appear to have an air of spurious importance. To patients who hold such views, the reporting of symptoms, such as a painless breast lump, growing mole or postcoital bleeding, is very difficult. They worry about wasting the doctor's valuable time or of appearing foolish. We know of one doctor who, when greeted by a patient with the words 'I hope I am not wasting your time' always replies 'I hope you are'! For people who feel like this it is important to offer alternative ways of reaching care. This is why the Birmingham experiments in the use of a nurse practitioner[1] have been so important, since they have demonstrated the value of primary consultation with specially trained nurses. Patients find discussing what they believe to be minor symptoms with nurses much easier. Medical critics of the use of the nurse practitioner hold that the evaluation of symptoms is very difficult and needs greater training. Though such an argument clearly has substance it is hard to see how a doctor can evaluate a symptom which he never sees because of barriers between him and the patient. As consultations in primary care are more with doctors than with nurses, much of this chapter will be directed at doctors. Even though the examples quoted relate to doctors the same principles can also apply to nurses.

The consultation

Everyone in the primary care team is important in establishing a proper diagnosis, made in physical, psychological and social terms. Receptionists who see the patient first may observe important evidence regarding how ill or disturbed the patient may be. The patient may offer facts indicating the reason for wishing to see the doctor or nurse and such information should, where possible, be passed on. A receptionist may also find out other important factors for example that a patient's near relative has just died, which should be passed on to the doctor.

Once the patient reaches the doctor or nurse, perhaps the most important factor is the allotted length of consultations. In Britain the average medical consultation lasts about 6 minutes. With nurses this is much longer. Studies in Belgium have shown that consultations with 'alternative' practitioners are much longer and this may be one of the reasons for their increased popularity[2]. A study in the Midlands[3] asked patients leaving the doctor whether they were satisfied that they had been able to tell the doctor all they wished to say. Over half the women between 15 and 45 years expressed reservations about this; the situation improved with increased length of consultation, being best when consultations lasted 10 minutes or more. In The Netherlands, mean consulting time with general practitioners is nearly twice that of their British counterparts[4] and a feature of Dutch general practice is an improved communication between doctor and patient. Of course it may be argued that there is not time to allow more than 5−6 minutes per consultation, but Dutch experience belies this, perhaps because it is possible to deal in one longer consultation with a problem that would otherwise take many shorter ones.

The whole ambience of the consultation is important. Care should be taken to ensure physical comfort, warmth, light and privacy. When the doctor or nurse and patient at last meet in consultation the carer's mode of greeting is important. Traditionally, the patient is summoned by bell or public address system and walks to the consulting room to stand knocking at the door as a supplicant. Such a start is hardly conducive to what may be a heart to heart talk; it is more like a visit to the headmaster's study in the expectation of six of the best! Once in the doctor's room, the doctor may be found with his head buried in papers while offering a grunt by way of greeting. Such a scene is fortunately now less common but still occurs. A better way would be for the doctor to get up and greet the patient at the door by name and with outstretched hand. Such a greeting shows interest and warmth and may help the patient verbalize his or her problem. Better still, would be for the doctor to walk to the waiting room and call the patient personally. This may be considered a waste of time, but that glimpse of the waiting room may provide clues about patients yet to be seen. In addition it is possible to observe the current patient, assess his or her physical and emotional state and, in the few seconds walk back to the consulting room, establish a friendly setting for the consultation.

Nurses often find this way of starting their consultations easier than doctors. It is interesting to note that in postgraduate discussions on the establishment of rapport in the consultation an increasing number of newly qualified doctors report that they fetch their patients from the waiting room. They sometimes add that it drives their reception staff mad!

Once initial greetings have been exchanged there is the question of where the patient should sit. Much has been said about the significance of a desk between the doctor and the patient and it is certainly easier for a patient to communicate when sitting beside the doctor rather than across a table. However, this is probably less important than the initial greeting. The importance of the relative positions of patient and doctor in the consultation lies in their ability to make eye contact easily and to appreciate and respect each other's body space and language. Body language is very important as a guide to the patient's emotional state—anxiety, fear, anger, sadness, etc.—and his or her gestures may have relevance to the symptoms described. The doctor may help the patient to describe his or her problem by demonstrating interest, leaning forward, nodding or offering affirmative grunts or ahs. Listening and being seen to be listening is very important, but so is watching. A doctor reported an incident when visiting a general practitioner friend in Norway where he did not speak the language. He was watching his friend during what was clearly a very intense and difficult consultation. In the middle, the Norwegian doctor turned to the Englishman and asked a question, then apologised for speaking in Norwegian and explained that he had asked for help in diagnosis. The English doctor replied 'but I know what is wrong with the patient, he is very depressed'. This diagnosis was rejected but 2 weeks later the Scandinavian wrote to his British friend and confessed amazement that without a word of the language the visitor had made a correct diagnosis. The moral is that one can be so busy listening that one does not see.

It is useful when a patient hesitates, or when there is a feeling of something left unsaid, to reflect the words of the patient back as a question, for example:

'I said to my husband . . . '
'. . . . You said to your husband?'

Similarly it is important to end with questions such as 'Have you understood what I have told you?' or 'Is there anything else you wanted to say?' Some British general practitioners, with the time constraints of practice, may find such communication devices hard to implement, but it is interesting that in The Netherlands very great stress is laid on just these points in vocational training.

In verbal communication it is important to use simple language that the patient can understand and to avoid medical jargon.

At the end of a consultation, it is useful to summarize the salient points as this helps to focus the patient's attention on them. Termination of the meeting is as important as the greeting since this will leave the lasting impression of the consultation in the patient's mind.

Medical men and women in hospitals may create artificial barriers of hierarchy, such as the ward round and even the white coat. If one watches an experienced clinician who is good at communicating you will see how he may circumvent these barriers by returning to the ward alone, in everyday clothes and by sitting on the patient's bed to give important information.

When giving bad or emotionally charged information it is important to be at the same level as the patient, sitting beside them or squatting or kneeling on the floor. Physical closeness is important and touch may be crucial in helping a person to come to terms with bad news. Some people find the establishment of touch difficult; this can be eased by starting with a formal handshake, or palpation of pulse which may then linger as a more emotionally supporting closeness. Sometimes the physical intimacy of examination may be useful in allowing a closeness of empathy between doctor and patient which may provide an opportunity for the exchange of emotionally charged information; while for others this may be the worst time since autonomy is only possible when completely clothed. The judgement of how to manage each individual requires great sensitivity. It is also important for doctors not to feel it is necessary to do everything themselves, there are many others to help: relatives, nurses, social workers, clergy and others. However, confidentiality must be respected and involvement of other carers must be with the patient's consent.

In giving bad news always find something positive to say, stress optimistic aspects of the problem, emphasize what can be done and how the team member and patient together will try to combat the problem. People can cope with the most incredible difficulties if they are given hope (i.e. any expectation greater than zero of a favourable outcome).

Lastly, it is essential to make records of all communications of important information and how it was received. This allows the whole team to know how best to help the patient cope. This is another function of the ONCARE card (see Fig. 16.2, p. 138).

References

1   Stilwell, B., Greenfield, S., Drury, V.W.M. & Hull, F.M. (1987) A nurse practitioner in general practice: working style and pattern of consultations. *Journal of the Royal College of General Practitioners* **37**:154–157.

2 Anonymous (1984) *Self Health* **5**:7−9.
3 Hull, F.M. & Hull, F.S. (1983) Time and the general practitioner: the patient's view. *Journal of the Royal College of General Practitioners* **34**: 71−75.
4 Tielens, V.C.L.M.G. (1987) *Consultations of general practitioners*. Thesis, Nijmegen University, The Netherlands.

Further reading

Byrne, P.S. & Long, B. (1989) *Doctors Talking to Patients*, 2nd edn. Royal College of General Practitioners, London.
Ley, P. & Spellman, M.S. (1967) *Communicating with the Patient*. Staples Press, London.

6 Control of physical symptoms: pain

Good symptom control depends on accurate diagnosis followed by the application of rational therapy. One is apt to become obsessed by the nature of the patient's cancer, but this is often irrelevant in diagnosing the cause of symptoms, except where sites of metastases in assocation with specific tumours or particular metabolic upsets are concerned. So the first question must always be 'What is causing this symptom?' Quite often the answer will be that it is due to medication. So the first cause may be the doctor who wrote the prescription. Since a patient may have several symptoms, even several pains, at a single time, this question needs to be asked of each one.

Pain is present in some 70% of cancer patients. It is an extremely complex symptom and difficult to define. One definition is 'an unpleasant sensory and emotional experience associated with actual or potential tissue damage'. Perhaps the most satisfactory definition is 'that which the patient says he is in'. Pain is a totally inadequate word to describe the suffering of patients with advanced cancer who are facing death, loss of their body image, bereavement from loved ones and ambition. It may be complicated by depression, loss of religious faith and anger at God or, more often, the doctor. In addition there may be physical pain of many different qualities and quantities. There are also preventable pains such as hunger, constipation, flatulence, urinary difficulties and mouth problems due to lack of oral hygiene. All this may be expressed as pain; perhaps anguish (which, like angina, derives from old French *angoisse*, choking) is a better word.

Pain perception may vary with cultural attitudes; perhaps the most extreme case is provided by the Navajo Indians whose language is the only one to lack a word for pain. Pain thresholds vary between individuals and with varying physical factors such as heat or cold, it may also be modulated by the patients emotional state. Many of us will have experienced trauma while playing sport which we have hardly noticed. The same degree of trauma when sad or not pleasurably distracted would have been severely painful. The gate theory of pain perception (Fig. 6.1) attempts to explain this. Neural mechanisms in the posterior root ganglia of the spinal cord act like a gate opening or shutting, increasing or decreasing the level of pain impulse which is transmitted to the brain. This effect occurs at the synapse between the peripheral sensory nerve and the ascending fibre in the substantia gelatinosa of the posterior horn. The ascending fibre then crosses the cord to join the contralateral spinothalamic tract carrying the pain sensation to the brain. The perception of pain within the synapses in the substantia gelatinosa is thought to be modified by inhibitory and excitatory impulses influenced from higher centres.

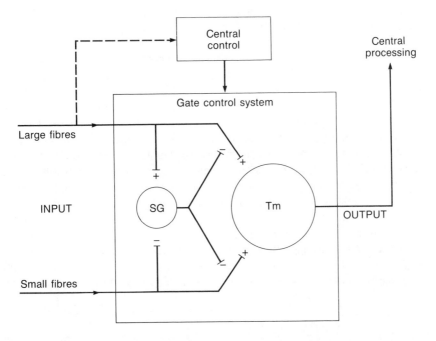

Fig. 6.1   The gate theory of pain perception. Large and small nerve fibres conduct stimuli to the posterior horn of the cord where there is a synapse with a transmission cell (Tm). A secondary synapse in the substantia gelatinosa (SG) exerts inhibitory and enhancing effects. The gate control theory postulates the opening and shutting of the gate by means of the increasing and decreasing effect of the secondary synapse. This in turn is influenced by mood, emotion and distraction of higher centres. From Twycross & Lack.[1]

The juice of the poppy *Papaver somniferum* has long been known for its opium from which morphine can be purified. Morphine has an extremely powerful pain-relieving quality. One wonders how this was discovered, somewhere in the mists of antiquity, for the idea that poppy juice should yield one of mankind's greatest balms is bizarre. This oddity became even more apparent when an antidote to morphine was discovered. This drug, naloxone, blocks the effect of morphine. Chemists, puzzling over the effect of naloxone, theorized a concept of key and keyhole where both morphine and naloxone are keys. Naloxone appears to fit the keyhole better than morphine and once the naloxone key is in the keyhole the morphine key cannot be inserted. The logical extension of this idea led scientists to wonder why the keyhole was there in the first place, and it was hypothesized that there must be a naturally occurring key. A group of polypeptide neurotransmitters were discovered which fitted the 'keyhole' exactly and which were infinitely more effective pain killers than morphine.

These substances were christened *endo*genous mor*phines*, later shortened to endorphins. The mystery of the opium poppy is partly cleared: by chance it has components that have similar key-like properties to the endorphins. Endorphin theory also helps to explain a number of bizarre observations about pain, including the dulling of its perception by distracting factors such as excitement or exacerbation by sadness. The idea that somehow one's endorphin mechanisms may be turned on by outside stimuli allows the logical explanation of pain relief through suggestion, hypnosis, the placebo effect or the many forms of alternative therapy. This concept will be explored further in chapter 11.

Endorphin theory also helps to explain why morphine does not depress the respiratory centre in the presence of pain. Once receptors, or keyholes, have been postulated it is easy to imagine these receptors opening up in the presence of pain. Morphine, prescribed in high doses for pain, does not depress the respiratory centre yet, in the absence of pain, the same dose may cause death through respiratory inhibition. This becomes important when a source of pain is removed (as may happen when neurological pain is relieved by nerve block). Under such circumstances if the previously required dose of morphine is not reduced following a successful block then marked toxic effects of the drug will be seen.

Causes of pain

Pain occurs with varying frequency in different cancers and is present most commonly in cancers affecting bone, the cervix and the mouth when it occurs in 80–85% of patients. At the other end of the scale, it is far less common in cases of lymphoma (20%) or leukaemia (5%). Pain is caused by a number of factors including tissue destruction, pressure, trauma, neurological involvement, muscle spasm, infection, ischaemia or disturbed metabolic function. Each of these may require a different method of control so a clear diagnosis of the cause of pain is required before logical treatment is prescribed. In addition, all of these causes of pain may be influenced by the patient's emotional and spiritual feelings.

1　*Tissue destruction* leads to the production of substances such as prostaglandins, histamine and bradykinins. This may occur with any type of destructive lesion but is particularly common in bone metastasis.
2　*Pressure* is a common cause of pain, as anyone who has experienced the pain of an abscess in a confined space (e.g. in the ear or under a tooth) will confirm.
3　*Trauma*, as may occur in pathological fracture, is painful in itself and also because of the release of prostaglandins from tissue damage.

4 *Neurological pain* may occur from direct involvement of nerves by tumour, as in brachialgia, sciatica or when an intercostal nerve is involved by a breast cancer. Neurological pain may also occur as part of a generalized neuropathy associated with malignancy or because of brain involvement leading to spasmodic pain similar to that of trigeminal neuralgia.

5 Pain may also arise because of *muscle spasm* particularly in the back and shoulders, where it is often related to anxiety or stress.

6 Cancers frequently become *infected* and this may be a cause of pain particularly in the head and neck, gynaecological and rectal cancers or in fungating lesions of the breast.

7 *Ischaemic pain* may arise because a large tumour has outgrown its own blood supply or because it is constricting adjacent blood vessels.

8 *Disturbance of metabolism* may occur with hypercalcaemia, uraemia or jaundice due to direct effects of the cancer, or may be associated with coincidental disease such as diabetes.

It is important to remember that many patients, particularly the elderly may have multiple pathology and that their pain may not be related to their cancer but to other conditions such as constipation or arthritis.

Pain relief

From the above list of possible causes it can be seen that pain relief in cancer may depend on the use of many drugs not normally indicated for pain relief. These include: antibiotics, anticonvulsants, antidepressants, and anti-inflammatory, antirheumatic, anxiolytic and spasmolytic drugs, as well as conventional analgesics.

As with all symptoms, the first step is to diagnose the mechanism of the pain so that the most appropriate measures for its relief may be adopted. Contrary to common belief, morphine or other opioids are not a universal panacea and some pain which will not improve with morphine will respond to other drugs. It is a safe rule to start with the simplest drug appropriate to the cause of pain at a low dose and then to increase the dose and relative analgesic potency of the drug until relief is obtained. The 'drug ladder' is shown in Table 6.1.

Table 6.1 Hierarchy of drugs for pain relief.

	First choice	Second choice
Non-narcotic drugs	Aspirin	Paracetamol NSAIDS
Weak narcotics	Codeine	Dextropropoxyphene
Strong narcotics	Morphine	Diamorphine

Different treatments are appropriate for each type of pain and do not necessarily involve the use of drugs.

1   Where pain is thought to arise from *tissue destruction*, for example in the presence of bone metastases, antiprostaglandin drugs such as aspirin or a non-steroidal anti-inflammatory drug (NSAID) will be the drug of choice.

2   *Pressure* may cause pain where a tumour is expanding within a closed space as in sub-periosteal or intracranial lesions. In such cases the reduction of tumour bulk by surgery, radiotherapy or steroids may be the best way of relieving pain.

3   *Trauma* may respond to immobilization, or where it is due to pathological fracture to surgical fixation, radiotherapy, NSAIDs or steroids.

4   Neurological pain may be due to pressure effects, direct nerve involvement or to a generalized neuropathy. Pain may be burning or stabbing in nature, the former may respond well to antidepressants such as amitriptyline and the latter to anticonvulsants such as carbamazepine or sodium valproate. The general peripheral neuropathy of carcinomatosis is more difficult but may respond to steroids.

5   The pain of *muscle spasm* may be effectively relieved by warmth, massage and anxiolytic and antispasmodic drugs such as diazepam.

6   *Infection* may cause pain by inflammation of the tumour or adjacent structures such as the bladder or pleura and may require appropriate antibiotics. The pain and discomfort (and also the odour) of infected fungating lesions may be improved with local applications of betadine or of metronidazole gel.

7   The pain of *ischaemia* may require tumour debulking by means of surgery or radiotherapy but where this is not indicated dexamethasone may be beneficial.

8   Where pain is exacerbated by disturbed *metabolic function* effort should be made to correct this (see hypercalcaemia, p. 65−66).

Opioids

Where pain is not controlled by the measures outlined above or by weak narcotic drugs such as codeine or dextropropoxyphene, then the next step is to progress to opioid drugs. Morphine and diamorphine are the most important, pethidine has little place in palliative care because of its short half-life which produces analgesia for 2−3 hours. Similarly, the synthetic opioid pentazocine (Fortral) has no place in the pain control of advanced cancer because it is a partial morphine antagonist, as is buprenorphine (Temgesic). Dextromoramide (Palfium) has a short duration of action and is useful as a booster analgesic before painful procedures such as changing dressings.

There is little difference between diamorphine and morphine apart from far greater solubility of the former and slightly greater potency. Diamorphine is extremely soluble so that it becomes the drug of choice when large doses are to be administered by syringe driver. The potency of diamorphine to morphine by mouth is 3:2 and by injection 4−5:2. Diamorphine is a semisynthetic derivative of morphine which is rapidly metabolized to morphine.

Rules for the prescription of morphine include:

1   Always give by the simplest route and simplest formulation, i.e. by mouth as a simple mixture of morphine sulphate in chloroform water.

2   Morphine produces analgesia lasting for 3−5 hours and should be given by the clock every 4 hours, *never* as required.

3   A patient's pain should be titrated with oral morphine mixture until the appropriate dose for analgesia is determined, it may then be appropriate to shift to other methods of administration of morphine, i.e. MST Continus (morphine sulphate tablets).

4   MST Continus produces analgesia lasting 8−12 hours provided they are swallowed whole. The slow release tablets should be prescribed two or three times daily and are available in the following colour-coded strengths:

> 10 mg golden brown
> 30 mg purple
> 60 mg orange
> 100 mg grey
> 200 mg aquamarine (a 400 mg tablet is expected).

Myths about morphine include:

1   In the presence of severe pain morphine in correct dosage does *not* depress respiration.

2   *Nor* does it cause addiction.

3   Though it may induce vomiting initially this is *not* a problem of continued use.

4   However, morphine *always* causes constipation so that concurrent prescription of aperients is essential.

Radiotherapy

Radiotherapy is a potent pain reliever particularly where pain is caused by bony metastases. The presence of spinal pain should always alert the carer to the possibility of cord damage and paraplegia which may be preventable with early radiotherapy.

Nerve blockade

In addition to the methods of pain control listed above it may sometimes be necessary to destroy pain pathways by nerve block[2]. These techniques are difficult and require the expertise of experienced anaesthetists to block dorsal roots, or the coeliac or brachial plexus. In severe pain when all else has failed division of the spinothalamic tract of the spinal cord may be considered. Where pain is relieved, as for example after surgical blockade of nervous pathways, it is important to reduce the dose of opioids. A patient whose pain was controlled on a high dose of opioid without signs of toxicity, may rapidly suffer respiratory distress if the dose is not reduced following relief of pain by nerve ablation.

Non-destructive pain relief can sometimes be dramatically achieved with transcutaneous nerve stimulation (TENS).

References

1 Twycross, R.G. & Lack, S.A. (1984) *Symptom Control in Far Advanced Cancer: Pain Relief.* Pitman, London.
2 Lipton, S. (1989) Pain relief in active patients with cancer: the early use of nerve blocks improves the quality of life. *British Medical Journal* **298**: 37–38.

Further reading

British National Formulary. British Medical Association and The Pharmaceutical Society of GB, London (published twice annually).
Doyle, D. (1987) *Domiciliary Terminal Care.* Churchill Livingstone, Edinburgh.
Regnard, C.F.B. & Davies, A. (1986) *A Guide to Symptom Relief in Advanced Cancer.* Haigh & Hochland, Manchester.
Souhami, R. & Tobias, J. (1987) *Cancer and its Management.* Blackwell Scientific Publications, Oxford.

7 Control of physical symptoms: gastrointestinal

Nausea and vomiting

After pain, nausea and vomiting are the most common and troublesome symptoms. They occur in about one-third of patients with advanced cancer. Again the rational management depends upon diagnosis of cause (Table 7.1). The vomiting centre and the chemoreceptor trigger zone lie in the floor of the fourth ventricle and may respond to a variety of stimuli.

Table 7.1 Causes of nausea and vomiting.

Primary causes	Secondary causes
Environmental factors	Cortical stimuli
Psychological factors	
Positional factors (motion)	Vestibular stimuli
Toxic effects (e.g. drugs/ cancer metabolites/ ureamia/ketosis/ hypercalcaemia)	Chemoreceptor zone ⟶ Vomiting centre
Physical factors (e.g. pressure on abdominal organs)	Intra-abdominal causes Raised intracranial pressure

Nausea and vomiting may be induced by any combination of five main causes (Table 7.1).

1 Environmental factors include heat and odours caused by strong sources of smell common to the sickroom, produced by excreta and the flowers or deodorants sometimes used to mask them. The common smells have been listed alliteratively as pee, pooh, puke and perfume and if this helps to remind us all that nausea is commonly caused by common things the mnemonic may be useful.

2 Psychological causes such as anxiety are very common. Just as hyperemesis gravidarum is sometimes relieved by removal to hospital with no other treatment, so the vomiting of advanced cancer may be settled by admission to a hospice and removal of stress in the patient's environment.

3 Positional, or motion sickness, due to vestibular upset is common and frequently distresses patients when travelling to hospital for treatment but may also occur when moving about their homes or getting out of bed.

4 Toxic effects are very common due to drugs, the cancer itself or to metabolic upsets such as uraemia, ketosis or hypercalcaemia.

5 Many factors within the gastrointestinal tract, for example partial obstruction, constipation, pressure upon the stomach and liver or distension may cause nausea and/or vomiting. Finally, direct effect upon the vomiting centre through raised intracranial pressure may be a cause.

Management

Often simple measures may be all that is needed: removal of strong odours or breathing through the open mouth may help. Sucking ice, sipping iced water from a wineglass, or drinking soda water is often helpful. The swift removal of used vomit bowls and the relief of anxiety by talking to and holding the patient may be very reassuring. Nobody enjoys vomiting and the preservation of privacy and the provision of attentions such as clean bowls, tissues and mouthwashes, do much to relieve the feeling of being antisocial so often associated with being sick.

Pharmacological management also depends on the diagnosis of cause (Table 7.2) with specific drug treatments indicated in Table 7.3. Where possible, drugs should be given by mouth; however, if vomiting is present this may not be tolerated. Domperidone may be given by suppository and hyoscine by skin patch. Dexamethasone, cyclizine, hyoscine and haloperidol may be given subcutaneously by syringe driver. Where vomiting is severe it may be controlled with subcutaneous methotrimeprazine (Nozinan) 25–200 mg daily by syringe driver. This is extremely effective but also acts as a very strong sedative. The synthetic drugs derived from cannabis, such as nabilone, offer considerable promise with regard to control of vomiting associated with chemotherapy.

Table 7.2 Causes of nausea and vomiting with anti-emetic management.

Cause of nausea and vomiting	Anti-emetic management
Cortical stimuli	Anxiolytic drugs, benzodiazepines, ? cannabinoids
Vestibular stimuli	Belladonna alkaloids, hyoscine antihistamines, cinnarizine
Chemoreceptor trigger zone	Dopamine antagonists, metoclopramide, domperidone
Abdominal causes	Metoclopramide, domperidone
Raised intracranial pressure	Dexamethasone* with an initial dose of 4 mg 4 times daily reducing to 4 mg twice daily

*Dexamethasone has many anti-emetic effects, possibly through cortical and emotional effects, appetite stimulation and reduction of pressure from tumour mass.

Table 7.3 Specific antiemetics and their indications.

Cause of nausea and vomiting	Anti-emetic of choice and dose	Side effects
Drug-induced causes	Haloperidol 1.5−3 mg at night *or* fluphenazine 1−2 mg twice daily	Side effects unusual at lower dosage
Radiotherapy	Prochlorperazine 5 mg thrice daily	
Chemotherapy	Prochlorperazine 5 mg thrice daily	
Metabolic causes		
Uraemia	Haloperidol 5−20 mg daily	May cause dry mouth or drowsiness
Hypercalcaemia	Haloperidol 5−20 mg daily	May cause dry mouth or drowsiness
Raised intracranial pressure	Dexamethasone 4 mg 4 times daily reducing to 4 mg twice daily	Euphoriant
	Cyclizine 50−100 mg 4 hourly	May cause drowsiness
	Hyoscine 300−600 µg thrice daily	Anticholinergic side effects
Intestinal obstruction (?caused by constipation)	Cyclizine 50−100 mg 4 hourly Hyoscine 400 µg thrice daily	May cause drowsiness Anticholinergic side effects
Oesophageal reflux	Metoclopramide 10−20 mg 4 hourly	May give rise to Parkinsonism
Delayed gastric emptying	Domperidone 10−20 mg 4 hourly	May give rise to Parkinsonism

Constipation

Constipation, like many other commonly used words is very vague. It is necessary to know what people mean by the term. To some it means failure of daily defaecation; to others merely a disturbance of a far less regular habit. Constipation may mean the passing of hard scybala or an inability to evacuate bulky soft faeces and, since these need different treatment, it is important to discover just what an individual means. It must be remembered that most patients are not used to discussing defaecatory function and may find it embarrassing.

Constipation is the most common preventable problem and often the most inadequately treated symptom of advanced cancer. Some 75−80% of patients treated in hospital or at home are grossly constipated. This may cause many symptoms such as malaise, abdominal pain or vomiting. Constipation is inevitable in palliative care unless it is prevented. It may result from dietary deficiency, reduced fluid intake (this is especially important with bulk-forming aperients such as bran), inactivity, gastrointestinal disease or, most commonly, as a result of medication with opioids. It follows that all patients receiving palliative care should have attention paid to their bowel function and all prescriptions for opioids should be accompanied by aperients.

There are four main causes of constipation in patients with cancer.

1   Reduced food intake, particularly bulk-producing roughage foods.

2   Reduced fluid intake or, possibly, loss of fluid through excessive vomiting or sweating.

3   Immobility which not only exacerbates constipation but prevents a patient from getting to the lavatory.

4   As a result of treatment, especially with opioids.

Management

Laxative drugs fall into four groups:

1   Bulk-forming agents: methylcellulose, bran, ispaghula, sterculia

2   Osmotic laxatives: magnesium sulphate (Epsom salts), lactulose

3   Faecal softeners: arachis oil, liquid paraffin

4   Stimulant laxatives:

   (a) anthracenes: senna, fig, cascara, danthron, docusate

   (b) polyphenols: bisacodyl, sodium picosulphate

A former proprietary favourite was Dorbanex liquid which patients tolerated well but which was withdrawn because of rare side effects; it is still available on a named patient basis for use in advanced cancer.

Since the patient may not be able to manage bulk-forming foods it is not usually appropriate to offer them and it may be difficult to increase fluid intake.

The first line of management is to perform a rectal examination on all patients with constipation. If the rectum is full of scybala it is not helpful to give bulk-expanding medicaments which merely convert the small hard lumps into larger softer ones which are difficult to pass. This type of constipation needs to be treated with arachis oil retention enema at night, followed in the morning by a phosphate enema. The patient may find this distressing but may be reassured by using soft incontinence pads to prevent accidents.

If, on rectal examination the rectum is empty and collapsed then there is no impaction. Usually this form of constipation responds to oral bulk formers and peristaltic stimulants.

If the rectum is empty but ballooned this indicates impacted faeces at the rectosigmoid junction; lactulose accompanied by either senna or bisacodyl tablets may be the answer. If the mass collects in the lower rectum this will need treatment with either a phosphate or micro-enema.

Rectal examinations to assess the precise state of impaction need to be continued until the problem is cleared. Once adequate bowel function is restored, all patients on opioids will require a maintenance dose of oral aperients. Lactulose 10−20 ml twice daily is the drug of choice and a stimulant such as senna or bisacodyl may be required as well.

Diarrhoea

Apart from the specific problems of palliative care for people with AIDS, diarrhoea is an uncommon symptom which occurs in only about 4% of patients with advanced cancer (unless they have concomitant bowel disease such as ulcerative colitis). One of the most common causes of loose motions is spurious diarrhoea caused by faecal impaction; this is easily revealed to the examining finger. Steatorrhoea gives rise to fatty offensive floating stools and is associated with pancreatic insufficiency. Diarrhoea may arise as part of a gastrointestinal upset, usually of viral origin, but may also be associated with a wide range of infections.

Diarrhoea is quite naturally distressing to the patient since it is exhausting and carries with it the associated anxiety about accidents and smells. This may be overcome if the patient is mobile, by nursing him or her near to the lavatory so that it can be reached easily. If immobile, then any call for a commode or bedpan should be immediately answered. The use of incontinence pads may give extra assurance but must be changed as soon as they become soiled otherwise the skin will become excoriated. If there is associated odour this may be best dealt with by the judicious use of fresh air rather than by trying to mask the smell with air fresheners.

Diarrhoea may be controlled with simple kaolin mixtures, though these are rarely adequate; sometimes sterculia, ispaghula or methylcellulose (used for constipation) will be helpful as they tend to bind loose stools and they may be particularly helpful after a colostomy or ileostomy. Antidiarrhoeal drugs which reduce motility are more frequently required. These include codeine phosphate, diphenoxylate (Lomotil) and loperamide (Imodium). Of these diphenoxylate may cause anticholinergic effects, especially dry mouth, and loperamide may cause rashes.

Faecal incontinence

This is an extremely distressing problem to both patient and relatives. The most frequent cause is simply due to the accident of not being able to be in the right place at the right time. Incontinence of faeces may be due to constipation, diarrhoea, the presence of cancer, neurological disturbance of defaecation, or to confusional states. In each case the underlying cause should be treated as far as possible. The most common cause after the one mentioned above is faecal impaction with spurious diarrhoea. This is frequently missed and needs urgent treatment (see above). Where no remediable cause can be found the help of a continence adviser should be sought. She or he can advise on aids and the most appropriate way of helping the patient.

Rectal symptoms

Rectal symptoms are common, embarrassing and uncomfortable. They may be caused by faecal leakage, infection or tumour. Faecal leakage or incontinence may be due to lack of sphincter control as in paraplegia, but may simply be due to spurious diarrhoea caused by constipation. Local perianal skin infection is often due to *Candida* and will settle with Canesten cream perhaps with added hydrocortisone. Rectal cancer may respond to palliative radiotherapy. Tenesmus is a particularly unpleasant rectal pain which is improved by chlorpromazine.

Halitosis and sore mouth

Oral symptoms are common and often not mentioned by patients. Drying of the mouth is frequent and may be caused by breathing through the mouth, infection with *Candida* or aphthous ulcers and drugs (especially cytotoxics and those with anticholinergic side effects). *Candida* is extremely common, and is probably found in 75% of patients, but is often overlooked. Bad breath can be very distressing to patient and carers and may be due to poor hygiene or disease, particularly cancer or infection of the oro- or nasopharynx. It may also be caused by disease of the bronchus (such as bronchiectasis or cancer) or to carcinoma of the upper gastrointestinal tract.

Management

Management depends on oral hygiene with particular care paid to dentures. The drying due to mouth breathing may be helped by encouraging fluids, sucking sharp-flavoured sweets or fruit, or the use of artificial saliva such as Glandosane. The use of lemon and glycerine mouth swabs every 2 hours may be very helpful. If the symptom is very disturbing, the patient's drugs should be reviewed and remove any unnecessary anticholinergic effects. *Candida* should be treated with oral nystatin suspension, amphotericin or ketoconazole. Aphthous ulcers may be helped by local application of hydrocortisone pellets. Halitosis due to delay in gastric emptying because of cancer of the stoamch may be helped by metoclopramide. The odour of oropharyngeal or bronchogenic cancer may be reduced with oral metronidazole.

Anorexia

Anorexia is probably more of a problem to relatives than to patients. It is very common in advanced cancer and often does not worry patients overmuch. Relatives on the other hand wish to serve the dying person and feel overcome with hopelessness as each tempting morsel is rejected. Sometimes canned baby foods will be taken when all else is rejected, and this may provide relatives with some degree of optimism.

Alcohol, in the patients preferred variety, provides calories, analgesia and may stimulate appetite. It should be served in appropriate glasses as a social event in the day rather than as yet another medicine. Many patients look forward to a drink long after other pleasures have faded, though how far one should go remains questionable. In one hospice, an old lady took some £150 worth of Courvoisier at the rate of a bottle a day in the last days of her life; she also denied she ever touched the stuff!

Drugs are rarely indicated for anorexia by itself, though when there are other indications steroids, especially dexamethasone, markedly increase well being and, with it, appetite.

Intestinal obstruction

Where possible, intestinal obstruction should be treated surgically. Where this seems to be unwarranted interference in a critically ill person then the condition should be treated medically. Often, where the obstruction is !ow in the gastrointestinal tract the evacuation of the bowel by enema may help enormously. If the patient can tolerate aperients by mouth Co-danthrusate may help. It may also be possible to reduce the obstruction by shrinking the tumour mass with up to 16 mg of dexamethasone for a few days and then reducing to 4 mg daily.

Vomiting should be controlled as much as possible, preferably with oral preparations, otherwise they may have to be given by syringe driver. First choice drugs are cyclizine or haloperidol, hyoscine may be useful as an anti-emetic but is very drying to the mouth. If all else fails to control vomiting then methotrimeprazine (Nozinan) may be given via a syringe driver but this acts as a strong sedative. Pain should be controlled with opioids or, if there is a great deal of spasmodic colicky pain, then antispasmodics such as hyoscine or propantheline should be used.

Loss of taste

Loss of taste may occur in advanced cancer and it is thought this may be associated with zinc deficiency which occurs in those on inadequate diet or in protein-losing conditions. Deficiency of zinc can be tested; the patient is unable to distinguish zinc sulphate in 0.1% aqueous solution from water. Zinc may be given as zinc sulphate (Zincomed) 220 mg thrice daily.

Hiccup

Hiccup is caused by diaphragmatic spasm leading to sudden inspiratory effort. Prolonged hiccuping, which may last for days, is exhausting, painful and humiliating. It may be caused mechanically, neurologically or chemically.

1 *Mechanical causes* include direct diaphragmatic stimuli from irritation by tumour or infection and by elevation of the diaphragm by ascites or hepatomegaly. A number of gastrointestinal mechanical effects may also cause hiccups including gastric distension and hiatus hernia.

2 *Neurological causes* include direct irritation of the phrenic nerve in the neck or mediastinum, commonly from involvement in a hilar lung cancer. Hiccups may also be caused by tumours involving the central nervous system.

3 *Chemical causes* are due to uraemia or to toxins from infection and occasionally from lowered carbon dioxide due to overbreathing.

Management

Treatment depends on the diagnosis and removal of the cause, but in advanced cancer these are often refractory because of the presence of the tumour or its metabolic effects. Stopping hiccups is not always easy. Many 'old fashioned' remedies such as drinking from the wrong side of the glass or cold keys down the back probably work, if at all, by reflex pharyngeal stimulation. Rebreathing from a paper bag is a simple means of correcting reduced CO_2 tension. Where there is gastric distension, antiflatulent preparations such as Asilone should be tried; metoclopramide may encourage gastric emptying. Chlorpromazine may be given 25 mg intravenously with a further 25 mg intramuscularly, but patients must be warned to expect drowsiness and lightheadedness. In very severe and persistent hiccups surgical ablation of the phrenic nerve may have to be considered.

Dysphagia

Dysphagia is commonly associated with cancer of the oesophagus or tongue but may also be caused by pressure from a mediastinal tumour or enlarged nodes. It can also occur as a result of neurological disorders such as multiple sclerosis or motor neurone disease, where the glossopharyngeal nerve is involved in tumour, or as a result of *Candida* infection especially in immunodeficient individuals (e.g. AIDS patients). *Candida* should be treated energetically with ketoconazole. Extrinsic pressure from a mediastinal tumour may be relieved by dexamethasone and obstruction of the oesophagus will require a Celestin tube. Inability to swallow causes problems with saliva and requires constant swabbing.

Because patients cannot swallow, it should not be thought that they cannot enjoy the taste of foods, even though the drink or food have to be spat out.

Squashed stomach syndrome

This occurs when the stomach is prevented from distending by the enlargement of the liver and may also occur where surgery or the tumour has reduced the size of the stomach. It gives rise to symptoms of fullness after a little food has been eaten associated with discomfort, flatulence, hiccup and nausea. It should be treated with carminatives (e.g. cardamom, Asilone) and metoclopramide to hasten gastric emptying.

Further reading

Doyle, D. (1987) *Domiciliary Terminal Care*. Churchill Livingstone, Edinburgh.
Regnard, C.F.B. & Davies, A. (1986) *A Guide to Symptom Relief in Advanced Cancer*. Haigh & Hochland, Manchester.
Twycross, R.G. & Lack, S.A. (1985) *Control in Far Advanced Cancer: Volume 1*. Churchill Livingstone, Edinburgh.

8 Control of other physical symptoms

Respiratory symptoms

Cough

Cough occurs in about a third of patients with advanced cancer and in 80% of those with lung cancer. It may be related to primary or secondary involvement of the lung with tumour, to infection secondary to the cancer, to concurrent disease such as chronic obstructive lung disease, asthma or bronchiectasis or to smoking. Many patients smoke long after their ability to enjoy other habits have gone. The cough may be dry and irritant or productive either with expectoration or pooling and swallowing of sputum. Dry cough is a much greater irritant to the patient and is often more difficult to relieve.

As with all symptoms a search must be made for the cause, which should be removed where possible. Bronchospasm will require bronchodilators by mouth or inhalation. Infection may require antibiotics. The underlying cancer may require treatment with steroids, chemotherapy and radiotherapy. Physiotherapy and postural drainage should be considered. Dry cough may respond to humidification of the atmosphere with steam inhalations or nebulized water to which salbutamol may be added if there is associated bronchospasm. Mucolytic drugs, such as acetylcysteine or carbocisteine, which have little value in treating non-malignant cough, may sometimes help those cancer patients who have very viscid sputum making expectoration difficult. Cough medicine may be helpful, though most simple antitussives are little more effective than steam or cough sweets which keep the mouth and upper respiratory tract moist. Where cough is extremely troublesome, the use of narcotic cough suppressants such as codeine, morphine or diamorphine as a linctus may be very helpful.

Dyspnoea

This is a very frightening symptom and tends to be self-perpetuating because fear worsens breathlessness. It occurs to some extent in up to half of all cancer patients and in two-thirds of those with lung cancer. Many patients express anxiety that they will choke to death or stop breathing while asleep and so struggle to keep awake. They should be reassured that neither will happen. Some dyspnoea is simply due to hyperventilation and will improve with rebreathing from a paper bag. Other cases may be due to remediable causes such as heart failure, asthma, chest infection or pleural effusion. For those with no remediable cause the most important therapy is listening, explanation and reassurance from someone who demonstrates a calm command of the situation. Simple measures such as sitting the patient up, opening windows, fans and breathing exercises may be helpful. Relaxation and some distraction such as reading or television may relieve the symptoms. In the absence of pain, morphine orally or, if necessary, subcutaneously, in small doses (2.5−5 mg) may dramatically improve dyspnoea by reducing respiratory drive. Anxiolytic drugs such as diazepam may help enormously. Oxygen, though often used, is less use than an open window. The patient may sometimes develop a severe panic reaction and the most effective therapy here is reassurance while the patient is held with a firm arm. Oral diazepam may be helpful but it is never as effective as calm supportive measures, including touch.

Haemoptysis

This is a frequent symptom of lung cancer and is often very alarming to the patient. Sometimes it is due to additional infection and may be eased with appropriate antibiotics. More often, it is caused by the cancer and is refractory to treatment. Patients require reassurance that they will not choke or bleed to death and may need sedation with diazepam or opioids. Rare terminal bleeding is dealt with in Chapter 15 (p. 124).

Central nervous system

Insomnia

Sleeplessness is common, occurring in 30% of patients with advanced cancer. It may be due to failure of treatment for physical distress, fear, anxiety or depression and should be discussed in depth with the patient. All the patient's physical symptoms (especially nocturia) and medication should be reviewed and treatment modified where necessary. Fear of not waking is so marked in some patients that they will fight to stay awake; here all that is needed may be reassurance and 'permission' to sleep. The patient's fears and anxieties should be discussed at length reviewing the psychological, social and spiritual aspects of their concerns. Particular attention should be paid to the presence of depression (see Chapter 9), which is suggested by early morning waking.

   When the above measures have been taken, recourse to drugs can be considered, bearing in mind that these may themselves have side effects and may further depress or sedate the patient. Alcohol may be a cause of insomnia where the individual has been accustomed to it and for some reason is not now taking it; it may also cause some early waking. Benzodiazepines may be very helpful, particularly short-acting drugs, such as Temazepam. Drugs with a longer half-life, such as Nitrazepam, though very useful in cancer patients have the disadvantage of producing prolonged sedation and poor daytime concentration. If this happens and the patient is at home, a second dose of Temazepam can be left by the bedside and taken if necessary during the night; the mere presence of the second dose is reassuring and often is not needed.

Fits

Convulsions may be due to pre-existing epilepsy or may be a manifestation of the cancer or its complications. They may be due to primary or secondary brain cancer or to uraemia. In undiagnosed individuals it is an indication for admission to hospital for investigation, but where the patient is known to have advanced metastatic disease cerebral involvement may be assumed without further investigation. Fits are extremely distressing for relatives and where necessary they should be warned of the possibility of such seizures and instructed in first aid for the patient. The immediate treatment is with 10 mg of intravenous Diazepam. If this is not possible, rectal Diazepam may be used. This is very safe and some relatives may be trained to use it when immediate help is not available. The tendency to fit should be controlled with anticonvulsants such as phenytoin, carbamazepine or phenobarbitone, and consideration given to the use of dexamethasone to reduce the mass of cerebral tumours.

Weakness

This is so common a symptom of advanced cancer that is sometimes difficult to remember that there may be other remediable causes such as overmedication, depression, boredom, lowered serum potassium, raised serum calcium or endocrine insufficiency especially of the thyroid and suprarenal glands. Patients complaining of weakness should have all these reviewed, though often none will be found to be responsible.

Lack of mobility and paralysis

The increasing debility of advanced cancer patients produces many physical, psychological and social symptoms—many of which have been discussed under separate headings. An increasing lack of mobility is common among these. Paraplegia due to spinal involvement is a common complication of vertebral metastases from breast, bronchus or prostatic primaries and occurs in about 5% of cancer patients. The first symptom is usually pain which may precede cord compression by anything from hours to years. Pain is usually felt at the site of the affected vertebra and may be worse on coughing or straining. There may be referred pain, paraethesia or weakness and disturbance of sphincter function.

The condition requires speedy diagnosis as it may be possible to prevent paraplegia with radiotherapy. Once paraplegia due to metastatic cancer has developed it is usually irreversible, though urgent decompression should be considered. The resulting symptoms may be helped by physiotherapy.

Vertigo

Vertigo occurs infrequently in advanced cancer but can be very trying particularly for patients travelling to hospitals for radiotherapy or chemotherapy or to hospice day centres. Motion sickness is well controlled with hyoscine but this may produce unacceptable drying of the mouth. Antihistamines, such as cinnarizine or cyclizine, may be useful but metoclopramide and the phenothiazines, which are so useful in other forms of nausea, are ineffective in motion sickness. True vertigo may occur in co-existent Menière's disease, in cerebral or eighth nerve tumours and following aural surgery. This may be difficult to manage by hyoscine, the phenothiazines and antihistamines, particularly cinnarizine, may be helpful.

Restlessness

This may be very worrying to relatives, particularly when combined with mild confusion, when patients may pick at their bedclothes (carphology) or throw them off. They may also try to get out of bed and fall. Often the cause may be found in acute discomfort such as pain, a full bladder or rectum and such a cause should be searched for and treated appropriately. Recourse to drugs should only be necessary after the removal of physical causes. Restlessness is so disturbing to relatives that it may lead to their inability to cope. Every available help should be provided including night care from Marie Curie nurses or the night watch service available from some departments of social services.

Confusion

This is a common problem in elderly or very ill patients whether they have cancer or not, and requires great care in diagnosis. Confusion may manifest itself in any combination of symptoms including lack of concentration, loss of short-term memory, disorientation in time or space, misperceptions, paranoid delusions, hallucinations, rambling speech, restlessness, aggressive or noisy behaviour.

Most of us will recognize having had some of these symptoms and fortunately it does not follow that one is necesarily confused to have one or more of them temporarily. Such physical impairment as deafness, anxiety or pain may mimic confusion and it is important to exclude these factors before assuming that a patient is confused.

Management of confusion depends on the identification and removal of cause wherever possible (Table 8.1). As with other symptoms there must be as much explanation to the patient and relatives as possible, with stress on the fact that the person is not becoming insane. Physical restraint should not be used and the patients misperceptions should be explained and allayed. Drugs are quite as likely to be the cause rather than the cure and should be continually reviewed with reduction of medication whenever possible. If there is cerebral involvement with the tumour then dexamethasone may help. Drugs such as haloperidol, thioridazine or chlormethiazole may help but should be reviewed early and withdrawn if not beneficial. Methotrimeprazine is very sedative and may be required in severe cases.

Table 8.1 Causes of confusion.

Unfamiliar stimuli	*Psychiatric disorder*
Too hot or cold	Depression
Discomfort in bed	Anxiety
Full bladder or rectum	Schizo-affective disorders
Pain, pruritus, nausea	Schizophrenia
Dehydration	
	Drug-induced
Change in environment	Narcotics
Leaving home	Phenothiazines
Changing bed position	Antiparkinsonian drugs
Loss of known ward neighbours	Barbiturates
	Digoxin
Metabolic disturbance	H_2-blockers
Uraemia	Benzodiazepines
Hypercalcaemia	Steroids
Hypoxia	
Hyponatraemia	*Drug withdrawal*
Hypoglycaemia	Alcohol
Hepatic failure	Opioids
Toxaemia of sepsis	Barbiturates
Deficiency states	Benzodiazepines
(vitamin, hormone)	
	Other cerebrovascular diseases
Tumour-induced	Alzheimer's disease
Systemic effect	Cerebrovascular disease
Cerebral involvement	Dementia, AIDS, etc.

Carcinomatous meningitis may occur in a variety of tumours including lymphomas, breast and lung cancers. It may produce a rapid deterioration with signs suggestive of meningitis, with clouding of consciousness, headache and cranial nerve palsies especially or the III, IV, VI and VII nerves. A recent patient was seen to lose her sight and hearing very quickly due to carcinomatous meningitis from a signet cell carcinoma whose course from apparent health to death was only 4 weeks.

Skin

Sweating

This is a common symptom of advanced cancer and may be due to overheating since many hospitals and hospices are far too hot. Bedclothes may be too heavy or of inappropriate material. Sweating may be caused by fever due to secondary respiratory or urinary infection but may also be caused by the tumour itself. An H_2-blocker (e.g. cimetidine 200 mg) at night may help. Excessive sweating may sometimes be relieved by paracetamol, non-steroidal anti-inflammatory drugs (NSAIDs) such as indomethacin or by small doses of a β-blocker like propranolol.

Pruritus

Pruritus may result from pre-existing skin disease such as eczema or tineal infection. Commonly there is a dry flaking of skin in advanced cancer or there may be macerated skin caused by incontinence. Drug reactions should always be considered and occasionally there may be psychogenic causes. The most common causes relate to the cancer, as in Hodgkin's disease or melanomatosis, or because the secondary metabolic effects, as in jaundice or uraemia. Management consists of scrupulous attention to skin hygiene. Highly scented soaps, talcum powder or lotions should be avoided. Itching may respond to simple measures such as keeping the patient cool. Washing is particularly important in uraemia when patients may excrete urea and bile salts in sweat. Patients' finger nails should be kept clean and short to avoid excoriation and infection. The source of itching may be the nightclothes which should be made of cotton.

Drugs are more often the cause than the cure of pruritus but may be needed in obstructive jaundice when it may respond to haloperidol, steroids, such as dexamethasone or stanozolol (Stromba), or to testosterone. Cholestyramine is unpleasant to take and not generally recommended. When all else fails for itchy skin rashes, a popular hospice remedy is cucumber liquidized in a household blender and applied to the skin.

Fungating/bleeding skin tumours

These are particularly distressing because of odour, pain or disfigurement. Hygiene is most important and lesions may be cleansed and dressed with hydrogen peroxide or 4% povidone-iodine compounds such as Betadine one part to four parts liquid paraffin. Charcoal dressings are sometimes helpful. Metronidazole may be very useful either by mouth or applied as a gel to the fungating lesion. Sometimes this is difficult and a mixture of metronidazole 0.8% in KY gel helps its application.

Capillary bleeding and fungating tumours is distressing and may be lessened by applying dressings soaked in 1:1000 adrenaline.

Decubitus ulcers

Care of patients' skin is of major importance since the acquisition of decubitus ulcers or pressure sores can lead to further pain and discomfort which, with good care, can be prevented. The old adage that you can put anything on a pressure area but the patient is as true today as when it was first used.

When the patient is first seen, an initial assessment of the state of the skin should be made, taking into account other physical factors such as mobility, level of consciousness, continence and nutritional state. Regular changes of position, at least every 2 hours are needed whether the patient is in bed all the time or sitting in a chair. Aids such as Spenco mattresses and cushions, sheepskins, waterbeds, ripplebeds or bubble mattresses are merely adjuncts to such position changes. Although these aids have an important role when correctly used they are only part of that care. Good handling and lifting techniques are also important in order to avoid shearing the patient's skin and subsequent sores. Nursing care must be evaluated and reviewed daily and even more frequently in severely ill patients. Sources of potential trauma, such as watches, rings and long fingernails should be dealt with.

Urinary symptoms

Urinary symptoms may be due to increased frequency of urgency of micturition or to detrusor instability. Bladder spasm may be due to concentration of urine particularly in patients whose fear of urinary symptoms makes them frightened to drink adequately. Concentration of urine also predisposes to infection, so compounding the vicious circle. Bladder symptoms are common and may be due to infection. In the catheterized patient this should be treated with urinary antiseptic washouts such as chlorhexidine, and in non-catheterized patients with appropriate antibiotics. Bladder spasm may respond to anticholinergic drugs such as propantheline, amitriptyline or terodiline but if the anticholinergic side effects are troublesome then flavoxate (Urispas) may help.

Retention may be due to benign or malignant prostatic enlargement, it may be drug-induced (especially by anticholinergic drugs such as tricyclic anti-depressants), it may have a neurological cause or it may be precipitated by a full rectum. Occasionally, retention may be relieved by immersion in a hot bath but the majority of patients will require urgent catheterization.

Urinary incontinence obviously affects the quality of the patient's life in an adverse manner. A priority of care for each patient must be to maintain and promote self-esteem, this is particularly so in caring for patients who have urinary incontinence. It is important to ascertain the reason for the incontinence and if possible treat it. Each patient must therefore be medically examined in order to exclude underlying pathology or inappropriate medication. Faecal impaction is a common cause in patients who are receiving opioids. This obviously needs to be relieved.

An assessment of environmental factors should also be made. If the patient is at home it may be that the toilet is difficult to reach, because of reduced mobility or it may be upstairs or even outside. The loan of a commode and/or urinals can help in such circumstances and may be arranged by the community nurse. The lavatory may be too low for a patient with limited mobility and the provision of a raised toilet seat and hand rails may help.

The patient, and for that matter the carer, may find it difficult to talk about incontinence to anyone because of its association with shame and humiliation. The members of the caring team therefore need to adopt a caring and sympathetic but very matter of fact approach. They need to be observant too since often the first intimation may be the smell of stale urine.

For some patients, incontinence may lead to their reducing their fluid intake for fear of 'accidents', whereas in fact this will only exacerbate the situation. An explanation should be given to both the relatives and the carer that concentrated urine not only irritates the bladder lining, leading to frequency and urgency of micturition, but is also likely to become infected which may increase the incontinence problem.

If necessary appropriate incontinence aids should be supplied after careful assessment. The aid of a continence adviser may be requested and most local authorities have access to such a person. The community nurse may be able to arrange to use the local authority laundry service if there is one, and arrange for the disposal of soiled pads.

It is axiomatic that patients should not be allowed to remain in urine-soaked clothes because this is demoralizing and will also lead to breakdown of the patient's skin, thus giving him or her the additional and preventable discomfort of excoriation and the potential risk of infection. Some of the commercially available pads permit urine to soak through so that the skin is not in constant contact with urine.

In the final stages of the patient's illness it may be kinder to catheterize the patient in order to prevent the upset of persistent wet beds, for male patients, a condom-type appliance may be useful.

Metabolic disturbance

Hypercalcaemia

Hypercalcaemia occurs in about 10−20% of cases of advanced cancer especially where the primary tumour is in the lung, breast or kidney. Multiple myelomatosis may also cause hypercalcaemia. These tumours give rise to the production of parathormone-like substances. Mild elevation of serum calcium up to about 2.8 mmol/l rarely causes symptoms, but above this patients suffer worsening of all their previous symptoms particularly nausea, confusion, pain and constipation. In severe instances there may be dehydration increasing confusion and coma. Above 3.5 mmol/l it is unlikely that any treatment will be helpful.

Mild hypercalcaemia should be treated by giving fluids and steroids (dexamethasone 4 mg twice daily); if this is not effective then sodium cellulose phosphate tablets (Calcisorb 5 mg thrice daily) should be given to bind calcium in the gut, but these should not be given if the serum phosphate is greater than 5 mg/dl.

In severe hypercalcaemia the decision to start active, unpleasant therapy may be difficlt and it will depend on the patient's general state and willingness to tolerate aggressive treatment. Mithramycin 25 μg/kg should be given by slow intravenous infusion. This acts by inhibiting bone resorption and so lowers the serum calcium.

Uraemia

Uraemia is a common late event in many cancers especially those affecting the urinary tract. There is often little that can be done for it but the complications of thirst, drowsiness, skin irritation and pericarditis may be troublesome and require symptomatic relief.

Further reading

Doyle, D. (1987) *Domiciliary Terminal Care*. Churchill Livingstone, Edinburgh.

Regnard, C.F.B. & Davies, A. (1986) *A Guide to Symptom Relief in Advanced Cancer*. Haigh & Hochland, Manchester.

Twycross, R.G. & Lack, S.A. (1985) *Control in Far Advanced Cancer: Volume 1*. Churchill Livingstone, Edinburgh.

9   Psychological symptoms

There are many psychological symptoms associated with severe illness. Some of these may be frankly psychotic or confusional and these usually have physical and metabolic causes and are dealt with under physical symptoms. This chapter deals with anxiety and depression.

Anxiety

Anxiety is present to some degree or other in almost all patients with advanced cancer. This may be due to the presence of unrelieved physical symptoms such as pain, shortness of breath, haemorrhage or nausea. To the patient, his or her disease is an entirely new experience for which there is no yardstick of normality. The carers do not have personal experience but their knowledge of what may happen is vital to the anxious patient. Once a patient has realized that he or she has incurable cancer, every new symptom may be attributed to the cancer and the patient may assume that the condition is worsening.

Anxiety may lead to overbreathing and a common vicious circle may develop due to hyperventilation. Overbreathing reduces alveolar CO_2 leading to panic and tetany. Rebreathing from a paper bag can produce a rapid and dramatic cure.

It is also very important that records should be made of explanations given to patients, as varying explanations of simple symptoms by different carers may confuse rather than help the patient. Thus, patients need listening time more than anything else followed by detailed reassurance about their problems. Sometimes it is very difficult, for instance if patients want to know what is going to happen to them and turn to their carers as experts in death and dying to ask about how they will end. Particular fears in this respect may involve choking, in those who are dyspnoeic, and severe haemorrhage in those who are bleeding. These questions can be particularly difficult where the carer believes the patients fears may be justified. Though one should never lie to a patient there is a case for being 'economical with the truth' under such circumstances. Fortunately, choking is very rare and much can be done to relieve it. Sudden torrential haemorrhage is also very rare but requires special treatment (see Chapter 15, p. 124).

Drug treatment of anxiety has earned itself a justifiably bad name since in the past it has often been found easier to prescribe anxiolytic medication than to listen to the patient and to explain. These drugs do, however, have a place in palliative care, but only after listening and counselling. Choice of drug will often depend on the patient's other medication because anxiolytic or sedative drugs such as phenothiazines or hypnotics may already be being taken. Sometimes it may be more appropriate to adjust the dosage of another medication rather than prescribe additional anxiolytics. The benzodiazepines are among the most useful drugs. Diazepam may be given orally, rectally or intravenously and is rapid in action but does tend to sedate. Lorazepam is available for oral or intravenous administration and Lorazepam tablets are absorbed rapidly sublingually. Probably the best anxiolytics are morphine and diamorphine.

Management

1 Listen attentively and be seen to understand the patient's fear.
2 Reassure about the patient's unrealistic fears.
3 Minimize those fears that may have substance but do so without belittling them, for no patient will be helped by their anxiety not being taken seriously.
4 Remove relievable physical symptoms wherever possible, especially hyperventilation.
5 Touch is most important when reassuring frightened people. In severe panic attacks the firm holding of a patient in the carer's arms may be very helpful.
6 Only after all the above measures have been taken should one have recourse to anxiolytic drugs.

Depression

Depression is difficult to define and classify. There are four main concepts covered by the term which may be represented as the corners of a triangular pyramid (Fig. 9.1).

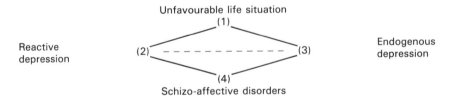

Figure 9.1.

A single patient may show any mixture of these concepts and so occupy any part of the space enclosed by the pyramid. Prevalence of depression in the total population is extremely difficult to assess and reports differ greatly between observers: much is unreported, much unrecognized and much over-diagnosed. Depression may be associated with physical illness to such an extent that it is suggested that as many as 25% of individuals with severe physical illness are also clinically depressed. On the other hand, the rate of prescriptions for anxiolytic and antidepressant drugs far exceeds the prevalence of disorders appropriately treated by them. Among patients with advanced cancer, probably the majority at some time show some symptoms of depression: this type of depression is usually of the first or second type though true endogenous depression sometimes occurs.

1 *Reaction to life situation.* Patients complain of depression and misery consequent upon unhappiness relating to their illness, disturbed relationships, or because of adverse social or financial situations. Such factors are common in cancer patients and may be contributory to, or exacerbate, reactive or endogenous depression.

2 *Reactive depression.* This is the depression caused by major, usually single, identifiable, personal disasters such as loss of loved ones, pets or property. Patients facing imminent death frequently grieve over their anticipated loss.

3 *Endogenous depression.* This form of depression wells up from within the individual, lacks identifiable causative adverse life events (though it may be associated with serious debilitating physical disease or major surgery) and is associated with self-criticism, anhedonia, a lack of future and suicidal thoughts, which in cancer patients may be expressed in a request for euthanasia. Endogenous depression is characterized by retardation of physical function especially bowel and sexual activity and alteration of sleep patterns with early morning waking.

4 *Schizo-affective disorders.* Severe disorders of emotion may be associated with disorders of cognition similar to, but falling short of, true schizophrenia. This is rare in palliative care except where the psychiatric condition was present before the cancer.

Pure forms of depression as described above rarely occur outside textbooks; most cases in practice present a mixed picture with a greater or lesser degree of anxiety or somatic complaints.

Depression may also be a side effect of anticonvulsants, clonidine, phenothiazine, methyldopa, reserpine and oral contraceptives. Benzodiazepines and other anxiolytic drugs may actually worsen depression. Depression is not just unpleasant; it has a small but significant mortality from suicide and there is increasing evidence of associated reduction in immunocompetence leading to increased risk of infection and malignancy.

Mechanism of depression

Considerable evidence has accrued in recent years to show that depression is probably caused by disturbance in the metabolism of neurotransmitters including noradrenaline, dopamine, γ-amino-butyric acid (GABA) and serotonin or

5-hydroxy tryptamine (5-HT). This metabolism occurs within the limbic system, an imprecisely defined collection of brain structures involving part of the cortex and sub-cortical nuclei. Depression is thought to result from cholinergic, and mania from adrenergic, predominance. Endogenous depression appears to be associated with altered functioning of serotonin (5-HT) in the central nervous system. There are multiple 5-HT receptors in the brain where it is thought antidepressant drugs may block serotonin uptake.

Management

Management of depression in patients with advanced cancer depends on assessment of the patient's position in the pyramid (Fig. 9.1). In all cases management involves listening, counselling and perhaps referral to social services and other agencies. Drug therapy is required in a minority who show evidence of marked pathological depression, usually of endogenous origin. Many forms of depression respond to treatment other than drugs. Treatment may include any, or all of: (1) simple psychotherapy; (2) social manipulation; (3) family counselling; and (4) drugs.

Suitable therapy for the four main types of depression are:

1 *Reaction to life situation*. Drug therapy plays little or no part in the management of unhappiness consequent upon a poor life situation. Listening and counselling, which are important in managing all forms of depression, and perhaps referral to appropriate social agencies are essential. Sometimes minor tranquillizers may be required in crisis, but anxiolytic drugs are *not* antidepressant and their use in undiagnosed endogenous depression may make it worse.

2 *Reactive depression*. Again, drug therapy plays only a minor role in most cases but antidepressants may be needed where the reaction is prolonged or fails to respond to listening and counselling.

3 *Endogenous depression*. Though the natural history of this condition is one of slow improvement, in palliative care it may markedly reduce the quality of the patient's limited expectation of life. Tricyclic antidepressants are the drugs of first choice though the newer tetracyclics may be indicated because of less side effects or cardiotoxicity.

4 *Schizo-affective disorders*. The use of antidepressant drugs may need to be supplemented with major or minor tranquillizers.

Drugs available for treatment

Tricyclic antidepressants are the most effective drugs in the treatment of depression and are of two main types:

1 Dibenzapines, including imipramine, desipramine, trimipramine, clomipramine, iprindole, opipramol and dibenzepin.

2 Dibenzocycloheptenes, including amitriptyline, nortriptyline, protriptyline, butriptyline, doxepin and dothiepin.

Of the two types of tricyclic antidepressants, imipramine and amitriptyline are the standards by which the others must be measured.

Choice of drug

Some drugs have an immediate sedative effect which may be very useful since many depressed patients are severely sleep depleted as a result of prolonged early morning waking. Dosage of tricyclic antidepressants is critical since there appears to be a relatively narrow therapeutic window, above or below which optimum response does not occur.

Anticholinergic side effects such as dry mouth, constipation and blurred vision may be troublesome especially in palliative care. Some drugs seem to have less effect in this respect and symptoms may be less marked if the patient is started on a small dose which is gradually increased every 3–4 days. A single dose given at night may also help patients to tolerate side effects. Because of their marked anticholinergic effects caution should be observed when treating patients with incipient glaucoma or prostatism. Depression in patients with heart disease should be treated with tetracyclic drugs (e.g. mianserin) which have a larger margin of safety.

Retarded and anergic patients may be helped by drugs with more stimulant action such as desipramine (Pertofran) or clomipramine (Anafranil).

Tricyclics may lower the convulsive threshold and must be used with caution in patients with fits.

Patients being started on antidepressants should be warned that the antidepressant effect of the drug will not be apparent for 2–3 weeks and that treatment may have to be for several months. Tolerance of anticholinergic side effects is improved with explanation to the patient. All antidepressants have a long half-life and can be given in a single dose at night when side effects will be less intrusive and insomnia helped.

Since the tricyclic drugs were first introduced a number of other antidepressants with slightly different properties have appeared. The tetracyclic drugs (maprotiline and mianserin) are structurally different from tricyclics and have little effect on cholinergic receptors and hence fewer side effects.

Monoamine oxidase inhibitors are less effective and more dangerous than tricyclics but have a small place in treatment; their potential usefulness is severely limited by their interaction with many foods. There may be interactions with other drugs, including tricyclic antidepressants, pethidine, phenothiazines, reserpine, sympathomimetics, antihypertensives and general anaesthetics.

Amphetamines were used formerly in the treatment of depression but their general use is now discouraged because of the risk of dependence or precipitation of psychotic states. However, they still have a place in the treatment of depression in palliative care. The risk of dependence in patients with a poor prognosis is small. This makes dexamphetamine preferable to tricyclics as its antidepressant effect is almost immediate. Despite disadvantages amphetamines may enhance the quality of life in patients with advanced cancer.

Steroids too have similar euphoriant properties and, though not advocated as treatment for depression, will be of beneficial effect when prescribed for other reasons.

Reference

1   Hull, F.M. (1988) The Management of Depression. In: Treatment in General Practice, Section 3.7. Kluwer Publishing, Brentford.

10 Spiritual symptoms

Everyone has spiritual needs and in times of sickness or great stress these become more prominent. Definitions include:

1 Spirit:

The force or principle of life that animates the body of living things. The fundamental, emotional and activating principle of a person.[1]

The singular concept defies definition. Denoting a form of being which has no distinctively material properties, 'spirit' (derived like its equivalents in many languages from words for breath or wind, as invisible, yet powerful and life-giving), connotes life, consciousness, self-activity.[2]

2 Spiritual:

Standing in a relationship based on communication between souls. Relating to the spirit or soul and not to physical nature or matter; intangible.[1]

Spiritual needs are very much to the fore in caring these days. Every nurse has it emphasized, both in the classroom and on the ward; but may not be helped to identify these. This lack of education is perhaps understandable in view of the difficulty of defining spiritual needs.

Miller and Keane define spiritual care as 'that aspect of health care that attends to spiritual and religious needs brought on by illness or injury.'[3] This puts religious and spiritual as separate entities.

The greatest danger in helping someone in need is in not listening or rather not hearing what the patient or relative is really saying. The tendency is for both nurses and doctors to say 'Send for the priest'. What they are not taught is *how* one recognizes when this is appropriate. Spiritual needs are not necessarily met by this method. In fact, at a time when the patient has identified someone to whom he or she can at last talk, they promptly abdicate all responsibility for meeting this person's needs by sending for a stranger. It is often only in a large general district hospital that there is a chaplain on call who can come quickly; as he may not be of the correct denomination the patient may wait for days which cannot be spared. It follows that attending to the needs of patients and relatives requiring palliative care is the responsibility of the person who identifies those needs.

Another trap which one may fall into, is that of automatically assuming that the patient is a lapsed Christian who wishes to return to the fold. This is compounded by the method of recording patients personal details, the space for religion is usually just the right size for entering 'RC' or 'C/E' and no more.

Many record clerks and nurses are upset if the patient does not want anything to be recorded, either because they cannot see the reason for anyone not having religious beliefs, or because they feel they must have every space on the record sheet filled. The patient either cannot see the reason for this question or immediately becomes worried that there is something he or she is not being told. The association of religion and death is quite clear to those who are seldom religious. Strange looks are sometimes given to patients who give the name of a minority sect as their religion: even stranger looks are reserved for those who call themselves 'atheist' or 'agnostic'. Atheists and agnostics (atheism: 'disbelief in the existence of any Gods or God'; agnostic: 'one who believes that God can neither be proved or disproved, and who accepts only material phenomena'[2]) are often people who have given a lot of thought to the subject and are secure enough to say how they feel. There are many who have not given spirituality any thought and, when confronted with the necessity of filling the space on the record sheet, lose confidence and reluctantly say Church of England. They may not have taken part in any church activities for many years and feel embarrassed by the question. All is not finished, however, as they may soon discover when confronted by the chaplain offering them communion.

The alternative is to say 'None' very firmly. This may be seen as a dangerous area since a patient may be worried that someone might try to convert them. A word of warning here for all qualified nurses: active proselytising could be considered a breach of the Code of Professional Conduct of the United Kingdom Central Council for Nurses, Midwives and Health Visitors.

How can we help someone in need to come to terms with the fact that their life is going to end sooner rather than later? The hardest thing is knowing when to keep your mouth firmly shut and *listen*. Listening means using one's whole body. Listening with the eyes may seem a strange notion but we often 'see' what people are saying to us, just as they 'see' what we say to them. Which brings us to our own body language: look at others and try to learn what they are really saying. What is the hidden message that is coming across? We have two eyes, two ears and one mouth, we should use them in that order and proportion when truly listening to people.

'Allowing', is a word that is used without its meaning being fully explored. Once again let us look at the dictionary since definitions of everyday words can be salutory, providing extra meanings which can enhance our knowledge and understanding and give us new words to use. Here are some of the meanings of 'allow': 'to pass, sanction, accept; to concede; to conclude, to permit, to indulge; to accord as due; to assign'.[4] We need to allow patients and relatives to *be*. Let us take another look at the definition of palliative care: 'That care provided for patients in whom, after exact diagnosis, attempts to cure have been considered and abandoned'.

These people know they may not have much longer to live. They need time and space to come to terms, not only with the knowledge, but also with themselves and the life they have left. This may be all too short, and they will wish to make the most of it. They need to consider the inner self, the Hindu word being *Atman* (self in us, the unmanifested ultimate reality, how we are inside). Being ill and unable to carry out the usual daily tasks often gives a person time to think and indulge in innermost searching, sometimes for the first time. What is needed is an ear to hear, someone who is listening with all their senses, without imposing values or being judgemental and who helps the patient's thoughts in words or pictures. The use of drawing, painting and poetry (other people's as well as the patient's own) to describe feelings can be used to assess as well as to treat. But probably the most important factor in spiritual care is the establishment of trust between the team member and the patient or relative. One must be aware of the barriers to achieving this. The main ones are time, privacy, space, language—having sufficient words as well as using understandable words. The 'KISS' principle (Keep It Simple, Stupid). When one feels ill or worried about a loved one it is very difficult to cope with long, obscure words and jargon.

Labun[5] in her article on spiritual care discusses O'Brien's seven examples of altered spiritual integrity. These include spiritual pain, alienation, anxiety, guilt, anger, loss and despair.

1 *Spiritual pain* Autton[6], describes spiritual pain as 'taking the form of belief that the pain or illness has been sent as a punishment from God for past misdeeds'. He also quotes Lamerton (1973) ' . . . the greatest pain of all, a pain of the spirit, is as great as mankind'. Believers may express feelings of discomfort or suffering in their relationship with their God as well as with fellow human beings. They may also feel they are lacking in fulfilment or empty in regard to religious meaning. They may feel unable to come to terms with their reason for being.

2 *Spiritual alienation* may cause feelings of loneliness, inability to see connections between past and present life and loss of purpose in being. There may also be inability to accept spiritual help.

3 *Spiritual anxiety* manifests itself as fear of the unknown, a feeling of impending doom. There may be a fear of meeting God, fear of punishment for real or imagined wrong doings. This anxiety may be influenced by attitudes acquired during childhood from religious teachings.

4 *Spiritual guilt* arises from concern about lifestyle. Could one have been a better husband, wife or daughter? The degree of this concern can enhance the pain of the spirit: 'if only I had done or not done so and so . . . .'.

5 *Spiritual anger* leads to the question 'What have I done to deserve this?' and may lead to searching for someone to blame: the doctor, nurse, hospital or religious institution. There is a feeling of being wronged or let down by those whom the patient looks to as 'saving' them from bodily and spiritual ills.

6 *Spiritual loss* is perhaps the most painful and concerns loss of faith in God. The stronger this faith was held, the harder it is to bear its loss.

7 *Spiritual despair* is felt at the loss of the love of God and doubt of regaining it when time is so short.

Altered spiritual integrity often manifests itself in somatic symptoms, especially physical pain, lethargy and anorexia, for which no physiological reasons can be found. It may be identified in discussion with the sufferer, though finding the appropriate words to describe it may be difficult. Few of us have sufficient vocabulary to say what we really feel. The team members need to be conversant with dictionaries and thesauri. Maybe use of the latter can help a patient or relative to describe their feelings. The carer needs to be secure in his or her own mind the precise meaning of words which are used, such as: pain, need, spirituality, beliefs, values.

When patients discuss their innermost fears it is helpful to ensure they are not interrupted. It is also helpful to ensure that the patient knows how much time is available for discussion. This is important as contact will be lost if the patient senses distraction, possibly resulting in him or her feeling guilty when there is already enough guilt to contend with.

There is a need to identify with the sufferer, involving one's whole being, sharing with others and having humility. The carer needs heightened self-awareness while trying to identify what is making the other hurt. The carer must be aware of the whole person and the interrelationships between stress and physical well-being. As with physical care, when the nurse or doctor should be wary of invading physical body space, so they should be equally aware of invading the patient's spiritual space.

How can the busy team member let the patient or relative know that he or she is receptive to the spiritual needs of the sufferer? How will the patient or relative know that the carer is receptive to his or her spiritual needs? This is where those little boxes on the patient's record might be of some use after all. They can be used as a discussion point, a beginning. 'I see you are down as being *x* religion, would you like to tell me how we can help you in your beliefs'. The problem is how to appear interested but not interfering; remember invasion of spiritual space can be as distressing as invasion of personal space.

Textbooks recommend moving conversation on to sensitive topics while carrying out a standard procedure, commonly a medical examination or bedbath. All very well for the fully clothed professional, complete with stethoscope and white coat, or plastic pinny and frilly cap. The patient barely covered by a thin sheet and having a cold wet flannel wiped over his or her intimate areas, is talked at whilst shivering damply. How can one possibly have a serious conversation with someone under such circumstances?

A more appropriate time is when both parties are warm, comfortable and clothed. Then the team member may quite naturally turn the conversation to deeper things, exploring what degree of observation or practice of religious beliefs the patient has by saying 'We do not wish to give offence so can you tell me enough so we get it right for you?' It is most important to record the discussion and to act on the information received. This way the patient will feel he or she has not wasted time and will be prepared to talk again.

Major religious practices

> Community is often defined by religious affiliation: One is a Moslem, Sikh, Hindu, Jew, Christian or whatever because of one's roots . . . regardless of beliefs or current religious practice.[7]

However much we dislike labels they can be useful points of reference when ascertaining degrees of observance or practice. It is impossible to be familiar with all the various religions in this country but a check list can be a helpful guideline to their basic principles. This will help you be aware of what you should ask.

The five main areas in the check list are: (1) religion; (2) food and diet; (3) hygiene and grooming; (4) medical/nursing procedures which might be offensive to the patient; (5) death and bereavement.

1 *Religion:*
   (a) Has the patient got a religion, what is the degree of practice/observation?
   (b) How will they wish to carry out such observation, are there any special requirements such as washing before prayer?
   (c) Is there a particular religious leader who may help meet spiritual needs?
   (d) Are there objects of religious significance and how should they be handled?

2 *Food and diet:*
   (a) Special dietary rules, proscribed foods, fasting.
   (b) Vegetarian, or special preparations?
   (c) If the relatives wish to bring in food, please remember that hospitals have lost Crown Immunity; check the institutions policy on food coming in from outside. It is suggested that such food is eaten only by that patient, all leftovers are disposed of safely. Food should not be left on the premises.

3 *Hygiene and grooming:*
   (a) Is there any special significance in clothing or jewellery?
   (b) Special care of skin and hair, shaving.
   (c) Bathing or shower.
   (d) Assistance by members of opposite sex.
   (e) Significance of right-hand/left-hand rules.

4 *Procedures and medication:*
   (a) Number of visitors, patient may wish to have more space available.
   (b) Female patients may prefer female doctor and male patients may prefer a male doctor.
   (c) Insulin from an animal source.

5 *Death and bereavement:*

(a) Which family member will assume the role of chief communicator, especially in non-English speaking families, what is the extent of their acceptance by other members of the family?

(b) The patient's wishes about the special preparations and procedures that the patient and family may wish to carry out.

(c) Their wishes about the postmortem, burial or cremation.

(d) Last offices.

(e) Expression of grief and mourning.

Principal religions

Judaism

One of the truly monotheistic (one God) religions which is not just a religion, but a whole way of life. The Torah, or law, is the light of the orthodox Jew's life. There are certain dietary restrictions which it would be useful to remember. Meat cannot be eaten which is not kosher, or fit. Offer only meat from ruminants with cloven hooves, e.g. sheep and cattle. Pigs have cloven hooves but are not ruminants and therefore not kosher. Animals need to be slaughtered ritually to be truly kosher. It is necessary to ascertain the degree to which dietary laws are observed. In any case it would be offensive to offer fish without scales, offal, or shellfish. Chicken is usually safe but meat must not be mixed with milk products in the same meal, there should be an interval of 3−5 hours between the two. Many Jews would prefer to be offered vegetarian meals if there is any doubt about the way the meal has been prepared.

The prayer, called the Shema, which is the first one a child learns and the last said before death, is said on waking and before sleeping:

Hear O Israel, the Lord our God, the Lord is One.

The Sabbath extends 25 hours, from sundown on Friday until 1 hour after sundown on Saturday. During this time orthodox Jews will do no work, not even switching off a light. This is a time for the family, usually spent in prayer, rest and relaxation. Many Jews value this corner of their lives as a time to think and to *be*. Letting the Jewish patient know you are aware of the Shema and the Sabbath and the importance of these in Jewish life, could enable you to become more helpful in meeting their spiritual needs.

Hinduism

Hinduism is one of the oldest religions recorded. It is monotheistic in that only one God, Brahman, is believed in. The apparent worship of many personal gods and goddesses is seen as one way for people to reach the Ultimate Truth, Brahman. As it is said 'there are many paths to the top of Everest, the important thing is to arrive'. Hinduism is one of the most tolerant religions.

The majority of Hindus are vegetarian. Remember taking the meat from a plate of meat and two vegetables does *not* make it vegetarian and would cause offence to many non-meat eaters.

Devout Hindus may pray three times a day: at sunrise, noon and sunset and washing before prayer is important. Modesty is important to both men and women. Women cover legs, breasts and upper arms, and men from waist to knee. It is vital that careful explanation is made before examining covered parts of the body. Hindus prefer to wash in running water and may consider sitting in a bath of water to be unclean. If a shower is unavailable they should be helped to pour water over themselves using a jug and basin. After defaecation paper is not used and the left hand is used for washing. The right is kept for eating. Handkerchiefs are considered disgusting because of nasal mucus, the nose may be cleaned with water which is expectorated.

Death to a Hindu is not a cause for sorrow. He or she knows that the soul is indestructible because of the belief in reincarnation.

Buddhism

Buddhism, in its purest form, is less a religion than a philosophy of life and a system of ethics. It originated in northern India in the sixth century BC spreading into Ceylon, Burma, Thailand, China, Korea, Tibet and Japan. Different sects arose in each country. The major ones are Mahayana and Theravada. Followers of the first, believe that no man lives alone and therefore his salvation must be involved with the salvation of others. In the second, it is believed that each individual must seek and find his own salvation. Buddhists believe in rebirth, the sequence of which only ceases for those who attain perfect wisdom and enter Nirvana.

In Britain there are many different schools of Buddhism whose festivals and diet vary considerably, although many are vegetarian. Customs of washing differ greatly; ideally privacy for morning and evening meditation should be provided. This meditation is usually done whilst sitting up, but can be done in bed when this is not possible.

Buddhists may refuse pain relief because of the importance of dying without a clouded mind. Careful explanation of all the effects of opioids should be balanced against the effect of unrelieved pain on the mind and clarity of thought. The patient may be offered a trial of analgesia so that he or she can decide whether to have further doses. Buddhists wish to be in control of their lives and to prepare themselves for death. They need close consultation about their disease process and treatment, and should have made their wishes known to their family or to a member of their order.

Islam

Islam, the religion revealed to Mohammad, means peace or submission. Its believers attain peace by obedience to its teachings. It is the fastest growing religion in the world and is militantly monotheistic. Muslims are committed to the code of behaviour contained in the Holy Qur'an (Koran) whose important terms include *haram* (not permitted by Islam) and *halal* (permitted by Islam).

A practising Muslim has religious duties called the Five Pillars of Islam:
1 Faith in Allah.
2 Daily prayer.
3 Fasting during Ramadan.
4 Giving alms.
5 Making a pilgrimage to Mecca.

Prayer is the essence of Muslim worship and every Muslim says prayers five times a day: after dawn, at noon, mid-afternoon, just after sunset and at night. These prayers consist of the opening verses of the Holy Qur'an:

> Praise be to Allah, Lord of the Worlds, the Beneficent, the Merciful, Master of Judgment Day, You do we worship and You we beseech for help; guide us on the right path, the path of those whom You have favoured, and not those upon whom You have brought down Your wrath and have gone astray.[8]

Muslims must wash and put on clean clothing before they pray, standing on a mat facing southeast to Mecca. The seriously ill are exempt from formal prayers but may pray privately, the carers should assist them but avoid overtiring already weakened bodies. They should be helped to wash as required.

During Ramadan, the ninth month of the Muslim year, fasting lasts for a full month. It begins at first light, when it is possible to distinguish between a black and white thread, and ends at dark. Devout Muslims may wish to fast even when ill and not take anything by mouth, injection or suppository. This may make symptom control difficult. In illness patients are exempt from fasting if it may affect the patient's recovery but exemption from prayers and fasting may be required from an Iman.

It is lawful for a man to observe fast on behalf of the other who is aged, awfully weak or dead.[9]

Islam holds that all males should conceal the body between waist and knees. Females should cover the whole of their bodies except face, hands and feet. Believers should refrain from wearing luxurious garments, which suggest vanity and conceit. It is unlawful for women to wear thin garments which show their bodies. Doctors should be the same sex as patients as physical contact between men and women may be seen as a sexual gesture.

The Holy Qur'an also lays down dietary restrictions. Food as well as drink used by a Muslim should be lawful (halal) and pure (tayyib).

Eat and drink and be not immoderate for Allah does not like the immoderate.[9]

Forbidden are carrion, blood and swine flesh. It must be ritually slaughtered, according to Islamic Law. If halal meat is not available then Muslims will eat a vegetarian diet. Alcohol is strictly forbidden.

Though Muslims believe that death is inevitable it is unlawful to be desirous of death. Only death can take the believer out from the world which is full of troubles, hence it is a gift to the believer. Death is seen as a temporary separation from a loved one. Special prayers are said for the dying: 'Allah, help me through the hardship and agony of death' is said to have been spoken by Mohammad in his last illness, he is also said to have prayed for forgiveness.[10] Other prayers include the declaration of faith 'There is no God but God and Mohammad is his Messenger', this should be recited by the patient, if possible when facing Mecca. Relatives and others will read to the dying from the Holy Qur'an. It is usual to say 'To Allah we belong and to Allah we return' when hearing of a death.

Sikhism

Sikhism derives from Hinduism and Islam. It was founded in the early sixteenth century by the Sikh Gurus, or Teachers, in particular Guru Nanak. It insists on the uniqueness of God, as with Islam. From Hinduism it derives its belief in rebirth. The way to salvation is through a good life, concern for family and society, and kindness to others.

Most Sikhs are vegetarians, some will eat meat but not beef. Sikhs are expected to rise early, say prayers at sunrise, sunset and before going to bed. Although there are no priests as such, many Sikh holy men are referred to as 'priests' for ease of identification. Sikh men have a duty to wear a number of objects at all times. These are symbolic and are often referred to as the 5 Ks:
1 *Kes*—uncut hair; none of a Sikh's hair may be cut. In an emergency permission should be sought from local Sikh leaders. Hair should not be shaved, but depilatory cream is acceptable.
2 *Kangha*—the comb, worn in the hair which is then covered by a turban.
3 *Kara*—a steel bangle.
4 *Kirpan*—a steel dagger; this is often in the form of a brooch or only a tiny dagger.
5 *Kacha*—white shorts worn as underwear, it is possible to shower and change these by keeping at least one leg in at all times.

Sikh women may sometimes also wear the 5 Ks. They are reluctant to undress in front of a male nurse or doctor and may actually refuse. They receive gold bangles on marriage which are as significant as the English wedding ring and should be treated as such. The belief in rebirth enables the Sikh to see death as not frightening. Many will receive comfort from hymns from the Guru Granth Sahib. The patient may read them him or herself, or a family member or a reader from the Gurdwara, the Sikh temple, may read them.

Christianity

Christianity is the religion which acknowledges Jesus Christ as its founder. He is the Son of God, the 'Word made flesh' (John 1:14). Their beliefs are summed up in the Apostles' Creed, which begins 'I believe in God the Father Almighty, Maker of Heaven and Earth . . .'. However, some sects prefer not to use it; among these are Quakers, Congregationalists, Baptists and the Plymouth Brethren.

Roman Catholics may derive comfort and consolation from visits from a priest who may administer the sacraments, particularly the Sacrament of the Sick. Privacy is important and every effort should be made to ensure this. Protestants may value a visit from the appropriate minister of religion. Holy Communion may be taken by those who wish. Patients may gain comfort from and ask for a Bible, a Prayer Book or Missal, a rosary, crucifix or prayer cards.

Many hospices have chapels into which it is possible for bedridden patients to be taken. This gives an opportunity for the whole family to worship together which may be a source of spiritual comfort to them. Every opportunity should be made for patients to be offered this facility, sadly few are aware of it. This means that a patient and family are denied this comfort and the team is missing a splendid opportunity to help ease the pain of separation.

Some Catholics and a few Anglicans may prefer not to eat meat on Fridays. Some may wish to fast or at least reduce or omit certain foods from their diet during Lent. All wish to have quiet privacy for their prayers. Facilities for hand washing should be offered before prayers, Holy Communion or the Sacrament of the Sick. The team should ensure that the patient is suitably clad when preparing to receive Holy Communion, Sacraments or a visit from a minister of religion. Some people may find it embarrassing to be clothed in night attire for such occasions; they may also not like to be in bed. The minister should be informed if a patient is particularly distressed by any of these factors. He may be able to help put them at ease.

Christians of nearly all denominations believe in an afterlife. Some can take comfort from the fact that they are to be reunited with loved ones who have died before. Some view illness and death, particularly if it is an early death, as a punishment from God and may feel guilty and afraid. This may be expressed as anger, either towards God or to whoever is nearest.

Humanists, atheists and agnostics

Humanists do not believe in God, preferring a scientific explanation for existence. They feel they are responsible for their lives on this earth and believe in mutual support and reassurance. Humanists see moral values as the principles upon which good human relationships depend. Such values include truthfulness, honesty, fair play, co-operation for the common good and caring for others. They believe that morality comes from within themselves, and in the finality of death.

Atheism is the disbelief in the existence of Gods or God.

Agnostics hold the view that one can never be certain whether God exists or not. There are many people described by Smart[11] as modern agnostics who simply do not attend church, temple or synagogue. They do not necessarily lack religious belief but do not feel they can belong to any organized religion. The formal worship of a God is not seen as an important part of their lives. As Smart says 'They see the heart of religion in loving one's neighbour, not in ritual'. Many have been alienated from religion by the rivalry between different faiths which they believe employ meaningless dogma. When encouraged to discuss their views they often refer to responsibility for one's actions, caring for others, the uniqueness of the individual and their right to their own religious and spiritual beliefs as their guidelines. Many of these people are worried by death, they may hope for an afterlife but cannot accept its existence.

All these people have spiritual needs, especially at the end of life. The team needs to take care in order not to upset the patient or relatives. One common worry can be easily allayed—that one must have a religious funeral. This is not so. There are humanist (non-religious) funeral ceremonies for those who wish, but prior knowledge is necessary so that the nearest humanist organization can be contacted.[12] Such funerals are normally conducted at a crematorium but can take place in a cemetery or elsewhere. The ceremony is a simple, personal one. Nothing is said that could offend anyone present who holds religious beliefs. This may alleviate fears about having a religious ceremony which may be felt to be hypocritical.

There are many pitfalls and many ways in which the unwitting team member can make mistakes and give offence. At a stressful time for both the patient and carer, it is easy for misunderstandings to arise. There is need for all concerned to be open-minded, sympathetic and honest, both with themselves and others.

References

1. *Collins Concise Dictionary*, 2nd edn (1988). Collins, London.
2. Hinnells, J.R. (Ed.) (1984) *Dictionary of Religions*. Penguin, Harmondsworth.

3. Miller, B.E. & Keane, C.B. (1987) *Encyclopaedia and Dictionary of Medicine, Nursing and Allied Health*, 4th edn. W.B. Saunders, Philadelphia.
4. *Chambers Twentieth Century Dictionary* (1977). Chambers, Edinburgh.
5. Labun, E. (1988) Spiritual care: an element in nursing care planning. *Advanced Journal of Nursing* **13**:3.
6. Autton, N. (1986) *Pain: an Exploration*. Darton, Longman & Todd, London.
7. Neuberger, J. (1987) *Caring for Dying People of Different Faiths*. Lisa Sainsbury Foundation Series, Austen Cornish.
8. Gaer, J. (1963) *What the Great Religions Believe*. The New American Library, New York.
9. Abdur Rehman Shad (1986) *Do's and Do Not's In Islam*. Adam Publishers, Delhi.
10. Brown, A., Rankin, J. & Wood, A. (1988) *Religions*. Longman, Harlow.
11. Smart, N. (1969) *The Religious Experience of Mankind*. Collins (Fontana), London.
12. British Humanist Association. *Leaflet*.

Further reading

Barnett, V. (1983) *A Jewish Family in Britain*. Religious & Moral Education Press, Exeter.

Cole, W.O. (1985) *A Sikh Family in Britain*. Religious & Moral Education Press, Exeter.

Cole, W.O. & Morgan, P. (1984) *Six Religions in the Twentieth Century*. Hulton Educational Publications Ltd, Cheltenham.

Harrison, S.W. & Shepherd, D. (1980) *A Muslim Family in Britain*. Religious & Moral Education Press, Exeter.

Ling, T. (1986) *A History of Religion East and West*. Macmillan Student Editions, London.

Ray, S. (1986) *A Hindu Family in Britain*. Religious & Moral Education Press, Exeter.

Sampson, C. (1982) *The Neglected Ethic*. McGraw–Hill, New York.

Sherratt, B.W. & Hawkin, D.J. (1972) *Gods and Men*. Blackie, Glasgow.

11 Complementary medicine, has it a place?

More than a million people in Britain now seek help from more than 30 000 alternative practitioners every year. The medical profession has even been requested by Prince Charles to re-examine its attitudes to complementary or alternative medicine. In an address when he was BMA president, he said 'when it comes to healing people it seems to me that account has to be taken of those sometimes long-neglected complementary methods of medicine which, in the right hands, can bring considerable relief, if not hope, to an increasing number of people'. It is therefore important to include complementary medicine in any discussion about palliative care.

Complementary medicine may be divided into several broad categories, all of which claim to involve the whole patient in his or her physical, psychological, social and spiritual totality. For this reason the term holism is applied. This may be criticized, since it is confused with the philosophical theory of General Smuts of South Africa who propounded holism in the statement 'The whole of man is greater than the sum of his physical, psychological and spiritual parts'.[2] The word holism is often used as a synonym for complementary or non-allopathic medicine, wrongly implying that holism is confined to those alternatives.

A BMA report[1] highlighted certain aspects of the alternative practitioner's art, he gave time, he touched his patients, he was possessed of authority and had a certain magic quality. These points are relevant. A study of the practice of alternative medicine in Belgium showed that patients felt its practitioners gave them more time.[3] In view of the average general practitioner consultation in Britain being about 6 minutes this may well be important. Touching patients is often a neglected means of communication and all must be aware of the import-ance of charisma, authority or, as it used to be called, bedside manner.

Philosophical approaches

Ayurveda

Ayurveda is probably the oldest known form of healing dating possibly from Mesopotamia as early as 3000 years BC and is the basis for Indian, Nepalese and Tibetan medicine. The name derives from the sanskrit words *ayur* (life) and *veda* (knowledge) and is more a religion and philosophy than a form of healing. It depends on the balance of three elemental forces which create, destroy or preserve and which are balanced by the physical, mental and spiritual state of the individual. This has something in common with the four humours, phlegm, blood, bile and black bile of Greek health concepts. Ayurvedic medicine seeks to cure through meditation, fasting, ritual and penance and it has given rise to much of the thinking behind many other forms of non-allopathic medicine such as homoeopathy and radiesthesia.

Anthroposophy

Anthroposophical medicine was inspired by the work of Rudolf Steiner (1861 – 1925). The name is derived from *anthropos* (man) and *sopia* (wisdom) and much of its philosophy depends on Steiner's *Philosophy of Freedom* published in 1894. Man consists, according to Steiner, of four bodies; the physical, the etheric or creative body, the astral body which contains his emotions and aspirations, and the conscious body similar to the ego of Freudian psychology. Again disease is seen as an imbalance between these bodily forces. Steiner would reject the modern concept of reductionism, which holds that if one can only reduce all problems to the simplest level of biochemical change then all will be revealed, in favour of a global view of man in all his bodies. Interestingly, he placed the seat of all these functioning bodies in the brain where, as we shall see, modern reductionist science is also focusing but with entirely different emphasis.

Anthroposophical medicine relies on many therapeutic methods including posture, movement, rhythm, music and painting to achieve the necessary harmony between the four bodies.

Complete systems of healing involving diagnosis and management

Acupuncture

Acupuncture depends on stimulation of areas of the skin by fine needles. It has been practised in China for some 3000 years but fell into disrepute during the Ching dynasty (1644 – 1911). Recently, it has again become more popular in China. Chinese traditional medicine depends on the balance between Yin and Yang; opposites of masculine and feminine, positive and negative, active and passive. The Chinese believe that these energies flow through the body in certain anatomically placed channels and that where there is imbalance between the forces illness results. Balance may be restored by placing needles in the appropriate channels.[4] Moxibustion is a variant of which small quantities of herbs are burnt over acupuncture meridia.

Herbalism

Herbal medicine is familiar to many of us as the major form of early Renaissance treatment. Indeed many aspects of it remain in use today—where would we be in our work in palliative medicine without the poppy? Many of us will have used the foxglove, deadly nightshade, curare, moulds, willow or cinchona bark. Even the contraceptive pill derives from the Mexican yam!

An extension of herbal therapy was advocated by Edward Bach (1880–1936) who was a pathologist and bacteriologist in the Homoeopathic Hospital in London. Dr Bach convinced himself that the sun-warmed dew of certain plants had very powerful healing qualities. The dew absorbed this quality and it was this that gave rise to the expression 'flower power' which was common in the hippy days of the sixties and seventies. Bach perfected a technique of absorbing this power by immersing petals in spring water in full sun for some hours.

Osteopathy

Osteopathy is a descendant of bone-setting which has its origins in antiquity. In its modern form it was founded by an American, Andrew Taylor Still (1828–1917). The theory of osteopathy is perhaps more acceptable to allopaths, and indeed many of its techniques have crept into orthodox medicine especially in orthopaedics and physiotherapy. In America, osteopathy is so well accepted that many medical schools open some of their courses to osteopathic students. The theory is that abnormal musculoskeletal function or somatic dysfunction, as it is termed by its practitioners, produces symptoms. Such dysfunction may produce metabolites within muscles such as lactic acid and excess potassium ions which exacerbate the original problem. Those of us who have developed strain through bad posture, work or anxiety can easily accept this notion.

Chiropractic

Chiropractic is another very ancient form of therapy. It is described in Egyptian papyri but then became lost until 1895 when it was rediscovered by Daniel Palmer in America after he dramatically cured deafness by cervical manipulation. Palmer's theory is based on the assumption that many health problems are caused by minor subluxations of joints, especially between the vertebrae. Chiropractic, literally hand manipulation, depends on returning joint alignment to normal.

There are obvious similarities between osteopathy and chiropractic, both of which may employ rest, diet and exercise in addition to manipulative treatment. When one considers how little orthodox medicine has to offer for certain kinds of back problem it is easy to see how these practices flourish.

Homoeopathy

Homoeopathy is much more recent and stems from the theories of Samuel Hahnemann (1755 – 1843) who believed in a fundamental principle which originated much earlier with Galen (130 – 200 AD) and was expressed by Paracelsus in 1658 as *similia similibus curentor*, let like be treated by like. This means that a substance—say belladonna—which can produce symptoms of fever, heat and rash similar to scarlet fever may be used to cure the very symptoms which it produces. The other important aspect of homoeopathy is the theory of dilution. Active drugs are diluted to such an extent that only the smallest traces are left—perhaps of the order of single molecules per litre. Imagine putting a drop of gin in a swimming pool, stirring well and taking a teaspoonful of water from the pool to serve as a cure for a hangover.

Diagnostic methods

Iridology

Iridology is a diagnostic technique used by many alternative practitioners and depends on close study of the structure and pattern of the iris which, it is believed, reflect the state of the organs of the body. This has become extremely fashionable in New Zealand.

Colour therapy

This depends on the theory that body cells emit energy of different wavelengths and some of this may be perceived as colour. An experienced colour-therapist is alleged to be able to see the colours an individual emits. Indeed some experts can do this with the naked eye, while others require sophisticated screens which cut out competing light wavelengths. Once deficiency is diagnosed, treatment is directed at correcting it.

Radiesthesia and radionics

Radiesthesia depends on dowsing or divining which has been used for finding water or minerals in the past. Expert dowsers can predict the quantity, quality and depth of underground springs with great accuracy. Radiesthesia adapts the practice of water divining to that of diagnosis. Radionics is an adaptation of radiesthesia in which the divining rod has been replaced by other apparatus. It is suggested that diseased tissue emits some sort of wave, perhaps akin to radiowaves, which may be detected and interpreted by a suitable instrument. All sorts of curious 'Black Boxes' have been invented to detect these alleged waves. In 1922, a committee of enquiry under Lord Horder demonstrated to the Royal Society of Medicine that something seemed to happen. The first 25 attempts at diagnosis were accurate giving odds of 33 million to one against chance. However this did not exclude the machinations of conjury. In America, a chiropractor by the name of Ruth Drown became extremely popular with the technique but in 1951 she was convicted of fraud despite the testimony of many of her patients. Proponents of the Black Box include members of the Royal Family and even some doctors have been puzzled to explain some of the results obtained by its use. However, it is hard to understand how one drop of blood on a filter paper or a single hair could produce any form of energy capable of storing complicated diagnostic information from other parts of the body. Certainly there is nothing to support the idea of radiowaves propounded in the original theories.

Therapeutic methods

Massage treatment

These rely on massage combined with other concepts of whole person care. Rolfing, a form of massage developed by the American Ida Rolf, depends on the theory that bad posture produces thickening in the major fascial plains of the locomotor system. The technique involves deep massage often with considerable force and it is claimed that many who are rolfed actually become taller. The treatment, like so much associated with the masseur's skill, also involves psychotherapy and this may be responsible for much of the claimed benefit.

Another form of massage is very different from rolfing in that it is given very lightly and only with the finger tips. This is Shiatsu from ancient Japan. It has much in common with the theory of acupuncture, which arose independently in China at about the same time, and involves stimulation of acupuncture points with the finger tips. It is sometimes called acupressure.

Reflexology

Reflexology has similarities with Shiatsu in that it depends on stimulation of the acupuncture meridia in the feet to produce reflex changes in other parts of the body. Another bizarre event connected with foot reflexes is observed in hypnosis. When a deep trance is induced in certain subjects it is possible to regress them in time so that they relive events of earlier life. Regression to infancy is possible and may be accompanied by a change in the Babinski reflex from the normal downward movement of the big toe to infantile dorsiflexion.

Aromatherapy

Aromatherapy, the treatment of symptoms by olfactory stimulation also seems bizarre, and yet many women use it either on themselves or others. Cynics may say that the use of perfume is aphrodisiac, or at least attractive, to the opposite sex. There can be no doubt that in some cases this is true: it is well documented that a male moth can track down his mate over enormous distance by reason of the pheromones that she releases. The queens of social insects, such as bees and wasps, control their workers by means of pheromones which they release into the hive or nest. The dilution that must occur when a chemical substance is released by a moth into the atmosphere which can still be detected by its mate, a mile or more away is reaching homoeopathic quantities. Perfumes from plant and animal sources contain a number of complex organic substances whose pharmacological effect is little known and whose messenger effect can only be guessed at. Anyone who owns a dog will have observed how inefficient the human nose is although it is obviously still an important means of perceiving information about the environment. Aromatherapy is an attractive concept and when one ponders on the smells of fresh coffee, or soil after rain, or of beeswax—to say nothing of Giorgio or Schiaparelli—one can see how one's well being might be influenced.

Naturopathy/clinical ecology

Naturopathy and clinical ecology are methods of harnessing the body's natural healing forces and depend on observations at least as old as Hippocrates. There are many ways in which therapists attempt to increase the *vis medicatrix naturae* (the natural medical way) of the ancients. The French psychotherapist, Emile Coué (1857–1926) produced the concept of 'self-mastery by conscious autosuggestion' and popularized the catch-phrase 'Every day I get better in every way'. Franz Anton Mesmer (1734–1815) believed that everything was influenced by the magnetic fields which pervade the earth and made great capital out of what he called 'animal magnetism'. Both Coué and Mesmer depended on mental or hypnotic reinforcement of natural healing processes and indeed most of the practices already described (including allopathy) rely on many methods of enhancing natural healing. Naturopathy and clinical ecology depend on the removal of harmful stimuli from our environment. There is a lot of good, green, commonsense about that. However the theory that *all* disease is due to food or chemical sensitivity destroys the credibility that some of it may be.

Quackery

The word quack derives from the older German word *quacksalver* which was applied to a boastful physician who profited by the gullibility of humanity by selling them useless remedies for diseases he had usually invented. These often sounded pretty terrifying such 'glimmering of the gizzard, quavering of the kidneys and the wambling trot' from which all of us would no doubt wish deliverance! These alternative practitioners are less common since the nineteenth century, but not all quacks are necessarily charlatans, some are within the medical profession and actually believe what they are doing. Perhaps we have all indulged in a little innocent quackery at some time or other. One such gentleman in about 1750 discovered a novel use for the caecum of a lamb which helped to protect against syphilis. Instead of earning fame he became such a laughing stock that he was obliged to change his name by deed poll. Poor Mr Condom, just think how proud and rich he would have been today.

Does complementary medicine work?

In the last part of this chapter some of the evidence for and against the claims of alternative medicine will be reviewed. Perhaps this is best done by discussing whether it works, if it does, how does it, and lastly, should we use it?

The philosopher Joad always used to approach a question such as 'does it work' with the disclaimer 'it depends what you mean by work'. If one means do people sometimes benefit the answer must be yes, but whether they improve in the manner alleged is quite different. The precise relationship of cause to effect is always difficult to ascertain, as was made clear by Ambroise Paré, the sixteenth century French military surgeon and inventor of arterial ligation. Paré, on being congratulated on saving a soldier's life remarked 'I dressed him, God healed him'. The same fallacy is summed up in the Latin *post hoc ergo propter hoc* (after this therefore because of this). Much of our disbelief in strange cures lies in our inability to explain things that seem beyond the capabilities of our five senses. But how effective are our accepted senses? The uselessness of the human sense of smell has already been alluded to, but it has also been suggested that the introduction of subliminal olfactory sensation influences human behaviour. In short we smell things we do not know we smell. If this is true of smell how much do we touch and not know, or see or hear without conscious perception?

In its scepticism, scientific allopathic medicine states that the advertised cures are in fact no better than placebo effects. Here lies the fallacy. We do not know enough about the placebo effect; it tends to be regarded as no more than chance. If, on the other hand, we accept the placebo effect as being a means of providing subliminal stimulus to our consciousness then it is possible to explain how apparently nonsensical measures may produce a similar effect. It is not the homoeopathic remedy, the meditation or the Bach flowers that cure our patients' diseases. This external show somehow stimulates physical somatic changes which relieve or even cure the diseases. Thus, it is important not to measure *against* the placebo effect but to regard the properties of a placebo with greater wonder.

How does complementary medicine work?

Perhaps, in view of our natural scepticism, we can only answer the question 'does it work' by attempting first to answer 'how can it work'?

If someone is overdosed with morphine the results may be reversed with naloxone. The receptor theory of how naloxone and morphine act is explained in Chapter 6. The original theory arose from work by Goldstein at Stanford in 1971 and was developed by Snyder and Pert at The Johns Hopkins Hospital in 1975. Later in the same year Hughes and Kosterlitz, in Aberdeen, isolated a substance from animal brain which possessed pharmacological properties similar to morphine. Having found this substance 'in the head' they named it *enkephalin*. Later research was to lead to the discovery of other similar substances, the endorphins. These substances offer far greater potential pain relief than anything we have today. For example, Oyama in Japan was able to show that patients in intractable pain were relieved by spinal injections of β-endorphin for up to 3 days. These endorphins seem to be naturally occurring pain modifiers. Pain is useful to us as a warning mechanism but in excess it is harmful and may distract us from guarding against common danger. So it seems biological sense that we should both perceive and control pain. Endorphins are released along with ACTH (adrenocorticotrophic hormone) in response to fear or in preparation for fight or flight which may help to explain why pain perception is reduced in excitement. Endorphins are detectable in the amniotic fluid of parturient women in rising levels as labour progresses. Endorphins can be produced by electrostimulation of parts of the brain, particularly the grey matter surrounding the cerebral ventricles, and it is thought that the remarkable pain relief produced by transcutaneous nerve stimulation (TENS) is mediated in the same way. Here is an explanation of pain relief from acupuncture, which is known to raise endorphin levels; there is also less convincing evidence that its effect may be reduced by naloxone. At least we have enough here to provide a rational explanation for some of the phenomena we observe and that makes belief a little easier.

Endorphins appear to be chemical messengers, like acetylcholine and noradrenaline, within the central nervous system. We have known of such messengers, called neurotransmitters, since Claude Bernard (1813 – 1878) and modern biochemistry has revealed many more, such as serotonin and dopamine. Possibly the pheromones by which insects communicate and control their social systems come into the same category.

It is now possible to think of some of the brain's function as a series of electrochemical mini-explosions triggered by neurotransmitters in response to stimulation from either within the body or perceived from outside it. We know some of these neurotransmitters but can only guess at the existence of others. They appear to be polypeptides whose potency and function is similar to hormones.

It is known from bereavement studies that loss may result in increased morbidity from such organic disease as infection, myocardial infarction and cancer. Such well-documented occurrences challenged belief when first mooted but these too may be explained in terms of the effect of neurotransmitters. We are well aware of changes in blood chemistry in response to emotional reaction to stimuli from outside the body, which are mediated by catecholamine substances such as adrenaline. There is now evidence that certain other blood functions may be influenced in a similar way as a result of presumed, but as yet unidentified, neurotransmitters. An interesting study in recruits to West Point Military Academy revealed an important link between stress and infectious mono-nucleosis.[5] This is hardly surprising to general practitioners and parents who have long known that glandular fever is seen in connection with examinations.

Studies in America have demonstrated that stress effects the immune system of students taking exams by producing significant reduction in natural killer cells and that this effect was even more marked where the students were lonely.[6] Though there is no clear evidence yet, this relationship is suggestive of some form of neurotransmitter which links cerebral and immune system functions.

So we begin to get a glimmering of how some of these strange things happen. What this should do is to open our minds to make us less ready to scoff at things that, in the immensity of our ignorance, do not seem explicable.

Should complementary methods be used?

The answer to this seems fairly clear. We should at all times do what we consider to be best for those who have trusted their care and lives to us. For a young woman with an operable cancer, allopathic medicine and surgery offer the best hope of cure. However, when that woman has widespread metastatic disease then anything which improves the quality of her life is good. If acupuncture, aromatherapy, the special diets of naturopathy, or meditation help improve the quality of life then there is no doubt that they have a place.

Patients turn from conventional medicine for many reasons. In some places orthodox medicine is unavailable or very expensive. They may have an incur-able disease and be clutching at straws or attempting to improve the quality of such life as remains. It may be that because patients pay for alternative medicine its effect is enhanced. Also patients exercise choice in alternative medicine and this may give them a greater feeling of control over their situation. Whatever the reasons, this increased popularity of complementary medicine has an important lesson for allopaths. If people are forsaking orthodox medicine this is because it is not meeting their needs.

This raises a fundamental and important question 'what do patients need?' The answer is clearly shown by the increasing success of alternative medicine—patients need a healer that they can relate to. We should remember Balint's suggestion that the most important force in healing is what he called 'the drug ''doctor'' '. Maybe this is the most powerful placebo of them all, certainly one may observe carers in hospices prescribing it all the time. This use of the carer's own personality was formerly referred to as the bedside manner—a now rather outmoded, yet still important phrase. Edward Shorter, an American Professor of History, has written a fascinating book on this subject in which he traces the history of the doctor−patient relationship over the last century.[7] Briefly, his thesis is that as doctors have become more powerful in their ability to intervene in disease processes so their relationship with their patients has deteriorated. We see an adversarial aspect of the relationship developing, first in America and now in Britain. Increasingly technological, mechanistic medicine is replacing the archetypal doctor who really cared for his patient, who had time to listen and respond as a human being. We need to return to concepts such as those of Schweitzer who said 'It is our duty to remember at all times and anew that medicine is not only a science but also the art of letting our own individuality interact with the individuality of the patient'.

References

1   British Medical Association (1986) *Alternative Therapy.* BMA, London.
2   Smuts, J.C. (1926) *Holism and Evolution.* Greenwood Press, London.
3   Anonymous (1984) *Self Health* 5:7−9.
4   Lewith, G.T. & Kenyon, J.N. (1984) Physiological and psychological explanations for the mechanism of acupuncture as a treatment for chronic pain. *Social Science and Medicine* **19**:1367−1378.
5   Kasl, S.V., Evans, A.S. & Neiderman, J.C. (1979) Psychosocial risk factors in the development of infectious mononucleosis. *Psychosomatic Medicine* **41**:445−446.
6   Kiecolt-Glaser, J.K., Garner, W., Speicher, C., Penn, G.M., Holliday, J. & Glaser, R. (1984) Psychosocial modifiers of immunocompetence in medical students. *Psychosomatic Medicine* **46**:441−453.
7   Shorter, E. (1985) *Bedside Manners; the Troubled History of Doctors and Patients.* Simon and Schuster, New York.

Further reading

Balint, M. (1986) *The Doctor, His Patient and the Illness*, 2nd edn. Churchill Livingstone, Edinburgh.

Lewith, G.T. (Ed.) (1985) *Alternative Therapies*. Heinneman, Oxford.

Ornstein, R. & Sobel, D. (1988) *The Healing Brain: a Radical New Approach to Health Care*. Macmillan, London.

Osterweis, M., Solomon, F. & Green, M. (Eds) (1984) *Bereavement: Reactions, Consequences and Care.* National Academy Press, Washington.

Salmon, J.W. (Ed.) (1985) *Alternative Medicines, Popular and Policy Perspectives*. Routledge, London.

Stanway, A. (1986) *Alternative Medicine*. Penguin, Harmondsworth.

Stroebe, W. & Stroebe, M.S. (1987) *Bereavement and Health*. Cambridge University Press, Cambridge.

12 AIDS: a special problem of palliative care

There has probably never been such a well-documented epidemic as that of the acquired immune deficiency syndrome (AIDS). Despite this it is difficult to identify where it actually started. The evidence from stored blood transfusion sera over the past decade indicates that the original change in the causative retrovirus appears to have occurred in Central Africa possibly as early as the late 1960s. This is no aspersion on Africa or its people, any more than the influenza attributed to Hong Kong reflects on that city; viral mutations have to occur somewhere and the site is in no way to blame. In retrospect, it seems likely that the first reported case of AIDS was that of Dr Grethe Rask, a Danish medical missionary who worked in Zaire. She became ill in 1977 and returned to her home in Copenhagen where she died of *Pneumocystis carinii* pneumonia. Although the protozoan *Pneumocystis carinii* commonly occurs in the human respiratory tract it seldom gives rise to illness except in severely immunocompromised individuals. At the time nobody understood Dr Rask's illness but with hindsight hers was probably the first recorded AIDS death.

Four years later requests to the Center for Disease Control (CDC) in Atlanta for the drug pentamidine, used to treat *Pneumocystis carinii* pneumonia, suddenly increased. By July 1982 the beginning of an epidemic was recognized, in the United States 471 cases had been notified of which 184 had died. By late 1984, 7000 cases had been notified worldwide with nearly 50% mortality. The doubling time for the total cases was about 9 months but has since slowed slightly to 11 months. However, by July 1988 the world notifications had reached over 100,000. Seventy-four per cent were reported from the USA, 13% from Europe, 12% from Africa and 1% from elsewhere. It is thought that there is very considerable under-reporting of AIDS especially from Africa. Estimates of true numbers with AIDS are put at 200 000−250, 000; those who are HIV+ are likely to be in the millions. In Britain by September 1988, 9242 individuals were known to be seropositive for the human immunodeficiency virus (HIV). There were 1794 reported cases of AIDS of whom 965 had died. Comparative figures with other countries become easier to appreciate when expressed in rates per 100 000 population (Table 12.1).

Table 12.1 Comparative figures showing numbers of HIV+ people per 100 000.

United Kingdom	2.5
United States	27
Zaire	60+

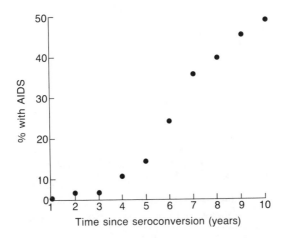

Fig. 12.1 Proportion of males developing AIDS by duration of infection.

Data from San Francisco suggests that progression from seropositivity to full-blown AIDS is variable and slow but that 50% of seropositive individuals will develop AIDS within 10 years (Fig. 12.1). Thus, if there were no more persons infected with the virus after September 1988, Britain may expect another 5000 cases of AIDS in the next 10 years. This is bound to be an underestimate since the known number of seropositives represents an unknown proportion of the real number of infected people and there is nothing to suggest that people have stopped becoming infected, though there is evidence that the rate of increase in infected individuals is slowing.

AIDS is still predominantly a disease of homo- and bisexual males (Table 12.2) though it is slowly spreading to the heterosexual population. Between June and December 1988 the number of HIV+ homosexual/bisexual males rose by about 11% while those believed to have been infected heterosexually increased by nearly 20%. It appears that an important bridge between these groups is made up of intravenous drug users. Blood and its products used in the treatment of haemophilia were a cause of early infection but are now safe. Concern has been expressed at the possibility of health care workers becoming infected by accidental needle-stick injuries. It is always difficult to be certain that sexual or intravenous drug routes of infection are excluded, but 26 health care workers throughout the world are reported as becoming HIV+ without identifiable non-occupational risk. When one considers the enormous number of medical and nursing personnel who have been involved in the care of potentially infected patients this number is minute. Seroconversion after accidental needle-stick has been estimated at 0.5%.

Though AIDS is now present throughout Britain it is still localized to major cities in England and Scotland (Table 12.3).

Table 12.2   AIDS in the United Kingdom, 30 June 1988 to 30 June 1989.

Transmission category	People with AIDS (%)						HIV Antibody Positive reports (%)		
	June 88		Dec 88		June 89		June 88	Dec 88	June 89
Male homosexual/bisexual	1315	(82)	1634	(82)	1927	(81)	4101 (47)	4545	N/A
Injecting drug user	54	(3)	70	(4)	94	(4)	1464 (17)	1576	
Receipt of blood/blood product	139	(9)	162	(8)	190	(8)	1149 (13)	1162	
Heterosexual contact	60	(4)	76	(4)	102	(4)	432 (5)	517	
Child of HIV+/at-risk mother	16	(1)	19	(1)	22	(1)	95 (1)	110	
Other/incomplete data	14	(1)	21	(1)	37	(2)	1553 (17)	1693	
Cumulative total	1598	(100)	1982	(100)	2372	(100)	8794 (100)	9603	10794

Table 12.3   Geographical distribution of AIDS/HIV in Britain mid 1988 to 1989

Country	HIV+			AIDS cases			AIDS deaths		
	June 88	Dec 88	June 89	June 88	Dec 88	June 89	June 88	Dec 88	June 89
England	7119	7833	N/A	1502	1863	N/A	852	1000	N/A
Wales	113	121		27	34		16	20	
Scotland	1504	1578		61	75		26	35	
Northern Ireland	47	51		7	9		3	4	
Channel Islands	11	20		1	1		0	0	
United Kingdom	8794	9603	10794	1598	1982	2372	897	1059	1272

World figures as reported to WHO at 1 July 1989

A total of 167,373 cases of AIDS have been reported to WHO from 149 countries but WHO estimates actual cumulative figures to be 480,000.
Cases reported:-

Americas		Europe		Africa	Asia	Australasia	
United States	95 561	France	6409	47 countries	24 countries	NZ	130
Brazil	6421	Italy	3773	30 064	373	Aus.	1334
Canada	2736	W.Germany	3324				
Mexico	2158	Spain	2296				
Domin.Rep	821	Netherlands	816				

The virus

The human immunodeficiency virus (HIV) was identified as responsible for AIDS by Gallo at the National Cancer Institute at Bethesda and Montagnier of the Pasteur Institute in Paris. HIV belongs to a group of RNA (ribonucleic acid) viruses known as retroviruses which possess an unusual enzyme called reverse transcriptase which allows DNA to be transcribed from RNA. The virus has the ability to insert its own genetic code into that of the nucleus of its host cell, so that the cell becomes a factory for the manufacture of more virus. A number of retroviruses are known, most of which affect non-human hosts. A retrovirus similar to HIV occurs in the African green monkey but does not infect humans. A new retrovirus HIV-II, which has similarities to the simian virus, is found in humans in Africa and there are some reports of its isolation in Britain. It may be that this variant accounts for some of the differences seen in the African epidemic which appears to involve heterosexuals more than in Europe and America.

Retroviruses are extremely fragile and easily destroyed by heating to 56°C for 30 minutes or by simple chemical disinfectants such as bleach. Although HIV has been isolated from many body fluids including saliva, tears, urine and faeces it is transmitted almost entirely through cellular contact between individuals. Such contact occurs in blood to blood or semen to blood admixture. HIV has a predilection for certain cells, notably T-lymphocytes, macrophages and glial cells within the CNS. Any fluid or tissue including such cells is potentially infectious. For this reason blood, and its products, or semen, which contains lymphocytes, are the most important means of transmission. Apart from transfusion and rare blood to blood contact such as tattooing, acupuncture or 'blood brotherhood' ceremonies, exchange of blood between individuals is rare. It does however occur between drug users who often leave traces of blood in their shared syringes. The most common form of transmission is still that between homosexual males. Anal intercourse allows semen with infected lymphocytes to enter the passive partners blood through tears in the rectal mucosa.

The clinical picture

Following contact with HIV, infection probably only occurs in a minority of individuals. Where seroconversion occurs it does so between 6 weeks and 6 months after infection and may be associated with a mild influenza-like illness often unnoticed by the patient. There may be no further development in some individuals or there may be a progression to the AIDS-related complex (ARC) in which there is chronic fever with night sweats, malaise and weight loss. At a later stage there may be persistent generalized lymphadenopathy (PGL). Progression from either of these HIV-related states may occur with the development of the full syndrome. The characteristic feature of AIDS is impaired immunity which manifests itself in opportunistic infection or unusual forms of malignancy. Opportunistic infections (OI) include many viral, bacterial, fungal and protozoan diseases which are normally rare in immuno-competent individuals.

Counselling of AIDS patients

Counselling poses additional problems because of the youth of many people with AIDS. The possibility of dementia (normally so rare among this age group) and potential cross-infection may give rise to special problems.

Counselling is complicated by the highly critical attitudes of society towards AIDS sufferers. This frequently gives rise to a situation where people with AIDS expect censure to such a degree that they see it where it is not intended. This became very obvious at a 1988 conference at London Lighthouse between general practitioners and persons with, or at risk from, HIV-related illness. It is sometimes very difficult not to be misunderstood and until individual carers are known and trusted, simple non-judgemental remarks may be taken as criticism and bitterly resented.

Counselling has two main aims: (1) to reduce the spread of HIV; and (2) to reduce the psychological effect of the knowledge of being infected with the virus. Education directed at avoidance of infection is a vital part of the preventive care provided by the primary health care team. It depends on education not only about AIDS, but also directed at changing societal attitudes towards the disease and its sufferers. Primary care teams should take every opportunity to increase the level of knowledge about AIDS in their practices, at individual consultations with sexually active patients, in schools and in women's organizations such as the Women's Institute. This is not to imply that the organization has any special risk, but because it is a huge nationwide group of women whose influence on the sexual education of young people is underexploited. The only real means of prevention lies in the alteration of sexual practices and the encouragement of monogamy, few sexual partners or safer sex. Safer sex has been widely adopted by male homosexuals in America and has resulted in a considerable slowing of the rate of spread of HIV-related illness among them. The risk associated with various sexual practices are shown in Table 12.4.

Table 12.4 Safer sex guidelines.

No risk	Low risk
Solo masturbation	Mutual masturbation
Non-genital massage	Dry kissing
	Body rubbing
Medium risk	*High risk*
Wet kissing	Anal or vaginal sex
Fellatio (if ejaculation does not	(without a condom)
occur into the mouth)	Fisting
Rimming	Sharing sex toys and needles
	Any sex act drawing blood

Fellatio = oral intercourse; fisting = insertion of fist into rectum; rimming = anilingus or insertion of tongue into rectum.

Counselling is also needed when there is a need for HIV testing. It is important to explain that testing for seroconversion is not a test for AIDS and that a negative test does not guarantee freedom from infection. It is also important to discuss the implications of a positive result before the test is carried out. A positive test only means that there is evidence of the individual having the virus and it gives no guide as to prognosis or to infectivity, however sexual partners should observe safer sexual practices. Unfortunately seropositivity will effect the individual, making it difficult to obtain life insurance and possibly reducing job prospects. In some cases it may prove difficult for HIV+ individuals to obtain medical or dental treatment. More severe effects are often psychological with anxiety, guilt, depression and obsessional illness.

Once any form of HIV-related illness is diagnosed, the counselling is similar to that of cancer except that patients tend to be younger and more prone to feelings of guilt and despair. Suicidal attempts are not uncommon shortly after patients are informed of seropositivity, though these often are less marked later in the disease when a more positive 'I will beat this' attitude seems more common. Initially, people with positive HIV tests show shock and disbelief which rapidly gives way to fear and anxiety about the future. It will be necessary to explore the individual's doubts and worries which may concern the course, treatment and outcome of the illness, rejection by society or sexual partners, or about the loss of autonomy and self-image. Patients may develop overt and covert depression, usually reactive, but which may be frankly suicidal. Patients may be angry at society, God, their sexual partners or they may be consumed with guilt at their own sexual or drug behaviour. They may also feel guilty at possibly having infected others. They may develop obsessional traits, either in a never-ending search for a cure, or with their own symptomatology. As with cancer counselling and communication, much therapeutic listening is called for with explanation and education about AIDS and reassurance stressing positive aspects of the individual case. As the disease progresses, counselling becomes more like that of advanced cancer.

Symptom control

The majority of patients with HIV-related illness are ambulant and as such are likely to be looked after in primary care. As the epidemic increases, therefore, there is likely to be a heavy burden on the primary care team. In very acute episodes, such as *Pneumocystis carinii* pneumonia, admission to hospital will be required and some cases may require hospice care. However, it is likely that most people with AIDS will be cared for in the community, as in America and those parts of Europe who currently have a high prevalence of AIDS.

Symptom control depends on cause which is usually due to opportunistic infections. The incidence of diseases in AIDS patients is given in Table 12.5, while Table 12.6 lists the cause of the different symptoms.

Table 12.5 Incidence of diseases occurring in AIDS patients.*

Pneumocystis carinii pneumonia	63%
Kaposi's sarcoma	24%
Candidiasis	14%
Cytomegalovirus infection	7%
Cryptococcosis	7%
Chronic herpes simplex	4%
Cryptosporidiosis	4%
Toxoplasmosis	3%
Other opportunistic infections	3%

*These figures are probably an underestimate since many patients have multiple infection.

Table 12.6 Common symptoms in AIDS and their cause.

System	Symptoms	Cause			
		Viruses	Bacteria	Protozoa	Fungi
Respiratory	Cough Dyspnoea	Cytomegalovirus Herpes simplex	*Mycobacteria* *Pneumococcus* *Haemophilus* *influenzae*	*Pneumocystis* *carinii*	*Cryptococcus*
Gastro- intestinal	Dysphagia High volume diarrhoea	Cytomegalovirus Herpes simplex	*Mycobacteria* *Salmonella*	*Cryptosporidium* *Isospora belli* Microsporidia	*Candida*
Central nervous system	Meningitis Encephalitis Dementia	Cytomegalovirus Herpes simplex Papovavirus	*Mycobacteria*	*Toxoplasma*	*Aspergillus* *Cryptococcus* *Candida*
Skin	All skin conditions are worse	Herpes simplex	*Staphylococcus*		*Candida* Tinea
General	Fever Weight loss Malaise		Consider all types of infection		

Respiratory symptoms

Respiratory symptoms are commonly caused by chest infections which may be viral, bacterial, protozoan or fungal. Respiratory symptoms may also be caused by pulmonary lesions of Kaposi's sarcoma. Bacterial infection should be treated with the appropriate antibiotic. Infections with atypical forms of *Mycobacteria* respond to normal antituberculous treatment. Pneumonia due to *Pneumocystis carinii* is treated with co-trimoxazole 20 mg/kg/day. As an alternative, pent-amidine 4mg/kg/day may be used. The majority (70%) of patients survive their first episode of *Pneumocystis carinii* pneumonia, but may succumb to subsequent attacks and a 2-year survival after the first attack is unusual.

Gastrointestinal symptoms

Gastrointestinal symptoms are very common, with high volume diarrhoea being the most troublesome. In many cases its cause cannot be identified but crypto-sporidiosis is among the most common causes, with other protozoan diseases due to *Isospora* or microsporidia as alternative diagnoses. Bacterial causes include *Mycobacteria*, *Salmonella* and *Campylobacter*. Where possible, the cause should be identified and treated, but often this is not possible. No reliably effective treatment exists for cryptosporidiosis. Parasitological and symptomatic cure of *Isospora belli* has been reported with pyrimethamine-sulphadiazine, trimethoprim-sulphamethoxazole, and furazolidone. Symptomatic treatment involves fluid replacement and drugs such as codeine phosphate or loperamide.

Mouth problems are extremely common, especially caries, gingivitis and ulceration of the fauces. Infection may be aphthous, herpetic, fungal or bacterial. *Candida* is especially common and its presence in the mouth of a young man is highly suggestive of HIV infection unless he is using betamethasone aerosols for asthma. Tongue lesions are common and hairy leucoplakia, seen as white flat warty projections on the lateral side of the tongue, is unique to those infected with HIV.

Dysphagia is common and often due to severe candidal infection which is often slow to respond to nystatin. In AIDS, *Candida* infection may be extremely severe affecting the oesophagus or occurring as a generalized infection with candidaemia. It requires aggressive treatment with amphotericin or ketoconazole.

Central nervous system

As many as 75% of people with AIDS show postmortem evidence of disease of the central nervous system, but only some 10% have neurological symptoms which may be caused by the virus itself, either because of opportunistic infection or because of tumours. About one-third of patients with AIDS develop a subacute encephalitis caused by HIV. In mild cases there may be forgetfulness and loss of concentration with lethargy and loss of motor function. AIDS patients may have several different HIV-related diseases and HIV encephalopathy may co-exist with opportunistic infection or tumours, as the following case history illustrates.

A South African homosexual known to be HIV+ arrived at an international airport unable to account for himself and was admitted to hospital. He was found to have neurosyphilis and widespread atypical tuberculosis as well as being HIV+. His dementia could have been due to any of his infections. While being investigated he developed frank haematuria and in his confused state was micturating over the walls of the general ward where he was being nursed. This caused great concern among hospital staff who wrongly feared infection with HIV from this source. Ultimately scanning showed the typical cortical atrophy of HIV encephalitis. After his syphilis and tuberculosis were treated he remained demented. —

Meningitis may occur in AIDS due to *Cryptococcus neoformans*. It is less florid in its symptomatology than acute bacterial meningitis but may resemble tuberculous meningitis. It presents with malaise and fever, headache with nausea and vomiting and there may be photophobia and neck stiffness.

Space-occupying lesions may be caused by opportunistic infections such as toxoplasmosis, or abscesses caused by *Mycobacteria* or *Candida*. Other neurological manifestations of AIDS occur as progressive multifocal leucoencephalopathy, a form of demyelinating disease, retinitis and peripheral neuropathy.

Treatment of neurological disease depends on treating the opportunistic infection where possible. Systemic fungal infection may respond to amphotericin, atypical *Mycobacteria* respond to standard antituberculous therapy, and toxoplasmosis requires long-term treatment with sulphonamides, clindamycin and pyrimethamine.

Skin symptoms

Almost all skin conditions become more florid in the presence of immuno-suppression. For this reason whenever one finds oneself thinking 'that is the worst case of (any skin condition) that I have ever seen' then one should also think of AIDS. All infective skin conditions, viral, bacterial or fungal, are particularly severe and require energetic treatment.

General symptoms

HIV-related conditions produce many non-specific general symptoms such as sweating, malaise, weakness, lethargy, myalgia and lymphadenopathy. These will require symptomatic treatment and treatment of underlying anxiety or depression.

Control of infection

It must be stressed that HIV is extremely fragile and is therefore difficult to catch unless there is blood to blood or semen to blood contact. Transmission may occur vertically across the placenta or rarely during breast feeding. This means that extreme care must be taken when handling potentially infected blood during surgery, venesection or in the laboratory. Blood suspected of being infected with

HIV should be sent to the laboratory with full biohazard precautions. Accidental spillage of blood should be flooded with hypochlorite solutions containing 10 000 ppm of available chlorine, and clothing contaminated with blood or semen should be autoclaved.

Tumours

The most common tumour is Kaposi's sarcoma which was originally described by Kaposi in 1872. Then it was a rare tumour seen in elderly Ashkenazim Jews. It has become more common since the beginning of the AIDS epidemic. It occurs more frequently in some groups of AIDS patients than in others, particularly homosexual males. In countries where the epidemic is more drug-than sex-related there are often fewer cases of Kaposi's sarcoma. Individual lesions may occur anywhere but are most commonly seen in the skin or mouth. They are multifocal and pigmented, often purplish or brown, and arise from vascular endothelium. Starting as a tiny skin blemish they rapidly develop and may be widespread.

Other malignant tumours include lymphoma and some forms of squamous cell cancer.

General management

As there is no cure for AIDS all care is palliative. There is some evidence that zidovudine (formerly azidothymidine, AZT) reduces mortality and morbidity in people with AIDS who have already suffered *Pneumocystis carinii* pneumonia or other severe opportunistic infection. The process by which reverse transcriptase encodes the RNA of HIV into the host lymphocyte requires thymidine, zidovudine acts by mimicking thymidine or inhibiting the insertion of viral RNA in the host cell nucleus. Zidovudine is expensive; treatment at 1989 prices costs about £120 a week or £6000 a year for drugs alone.

Other treatment must be supportive and symptomatic; there are many support organizations (see Appendix 2).

Further reading

Adler, M.W. (Ed.) (1987) *ABC of AIDS*, British Medical Association, London.
Adler, M.W. (Ed.) (1988) *Disease in the Homosexual Male*, Springer-Verlag, London.
Fischl, M.A. (1987) The efficacy of azidothymidine (AZT) in the treatment of patients with AIDS and AIDS-related complex, *New England Journal of Medicine* **317(4)**:185 – 191.

Greenspan, D., Pindborg, J.J., Greenspan, J.S. & Schiedt, M. (1986) *AIDS and the Dental Team*. Munksgaard, Copenhagen.

Hull, R. (1987) *Infective Disease in Primary Care*, Chapman & Hall, London.

Kaplan, M.H., Sadick, N., Scott McNutt, N., Meltzer, M., Sarngadharan, M.G. & Pahwa, S. Dermatologic findings and manifestations of acquired immuno-deficiency syndrome (AIDS), *Journal of the American Academy of Dermatology* **16**:485−505.

Knox, E.G. (1986) A transmission model for AIDS, *European Journal of Epidemiology* **2**:165−177.

Morbidity and Mortality Weekly Report, Center for Disease Control, Atlanta (1987) *Journal of the American Medical Association* **258**:1293−1305.

Shilts, R. (1987) *And the Band Played On*, Penguin, Harmondsworth.

Wells, N. (1987) *The AIDS Virus, Forecasting its Impact*, Office of Health Economics, London.

13   Care for the carers

Caring for the dying is quite naturally stressful and in any consideration of a teamwork approach the question arises 'who cares for the carers?' It follows that the carers' well-being is of optimum importance since if they are well, feeling confident and competent, then the patient will receive the highest possible standard of care. This chapter aims to explore the nature of the carers' stress and seeks ways in which this stress may be ameliorated or handled in a more useful way.

Stress is a common term and one with which we are all familiar but what does it mean? In reviewing the literature it seems to have developed multiple meanings which are often not congruent. Historically, the word is of Latin derivation first used in this country in the seventeenth century when it was used to refer to hardship or distress. Gradually, the meaning changed and was largely used in engineering where it was associated with strain. There have been many attempts to define the term, noteably Selye[1], Lazarus[2], McGrath[3], Jacobson[4] and Bailey[5]; and in looking at these it becomes clear that there is no definitive definition. A useful definition for this chapter is that used by Gaye[6]: 'stress is a perceptual phenomenon arising from a comparison between the demand on an individual and his or her ability to cope.'

How then can we help the carers, family member or professional, to cope with the demands of palliative care?

Unprofessional carers

The concept of caring is derived from the eastern Germanic *Kara* meaning to carry a burden with, suffer with, grieve and mourn with. Caring is always difficult, particularly so for the patient's relatives who are often front-line carers. When they are first acquainted with the diagnosis they will naturally feel shock and disbelief. This may be tempered by the hope that there has been some error in diagnosis. There may be guilt, 'if only I had got him to a doctor sooner', 'I should have noticed she was ill'. There is the distress of watching a loved one deteriorate physically. Perhaps this is the first time they realise their own mortality. It is often tempting for relatives to try and shield the patient from the knowledge of the diagnosis. This may be done to protect the patient or possibly themselves. These attempts cause greater strain, since often they lead to lies and distrust which can alienate the patient and the carer and may lead to breakdown of family relationships.

Since the family are usually intimately concerned in caring, it is obvious that they need to be involved in care planning. After all, they are the ones who know the patient best and they will constitute an important part of the team. If his/her condition permits, the patient too must be involved in this plan of care.

Good communication between all those concerned is vital and can help to assuage some of the stress. The family need to know what is happening and what can be realistically expected. Any communication needs to be at a level which they will understand, avoiding jargon and using familiar words. It is often helpful if the doctor speaks to the patient and relatives in the presence of other members of the team, since this ensures that each knows what the others have been told. It avoids any one member, particularly the patient, feeling isolated and can allay stress. For many people in today's society, death is shrouded in mystery. With increased life-span, it is possible that many in their thirties or even forties have no experience of death. The trend is also for more people to die in hospital. There is thus anxiety as they wonder how they will manage, and there may be fear about seeing a death; coping with the day to day management of such an ill person; worry about whether the patient should be cared for at home or in hospital. A sympathetic doctor can do much in this situation by setting out, and continually reviewing, the alternatives and the benefits each has to offer. Obviously, the patient's wishes are paramount. It can be of immense support to the relatives to know that the doctor will arrange for help and support in the home or a transfer to hospital or hospice when it becomes necessary.

Caring at home puts a strain on family relationships; the burden of care may fall on one particular family member, imposing physical, mental and emotional strain. The carer becomes tired, anxious and the patient may resent his/her loss of independence; there may be jealousies that one family member is getting more attention than another. All this can result in tension and irritability.

The support of a caring primary health care team is vital. A hospice may be involved to provide specialist assistance with pain control as well as the aid of a home care team of nurses who have been specially trained in aspects of palliative care. If the patient's condition permits, arrangements may be made for attendance at a day care unit of a hospice on one or more days a week. These units offer respite for the carer who thus has the chance to rest, or get away from the situation. For the patient they provide peer group support or, as one patient succinctly put it:

> Here you can come and be amongst friends. At home everyone is nice and they are really trying hard but they don't really understand what it's like (to have cancer). Everyone here knows, we're all in the same boat and we can support each other. They (the other patients) always know what I mean when I say I'm having a bad day—they've been there.

Whilst at the unit the patient can see the doctor if necessary, have a bath, beauty treatment and take part in a multitude of social activities. The atmosphere is more that of a social club than what is generally expected of a hospice. There is often a surprising amount of laughter. As one student nurse visiting a day unit for the first time put it: here the emphasis is very much on living.

Association in this way with hospice care can be extremely reassuring to the family. The courage and humour shown by patients supporting each other in a day centre may lessen the burden not only for themselves but also for medical and nursing staff.

Anorexia can cause the relatives much anxiety, since most of us equate health with eating. Simple explanations can do much to allay these anxieties. For example, a person who is not expending much energy does not need a big intake of food. It is axiomatic that if the patient is vomiting he or she will find it impossible to eat.

Incontinence puts added strain on the carer, who has to contend with the additional laundry and the distress of the patient. Clearly, it is important to establish the cause and if possible, treat it. The community nurse can arrange for the provision of incontinence aids, the loan of commodes, urinals and bed pans and in some areas a linen service may be available.

Financial difficulties are common and the aid of a social worker is invaluable since they may be able to arrange for assistance from a variety of sources, some of which are listed in Appendix 2.

One difficulty which carers, and for that matter patients, are reluctant to admit to are those associated with intimacy and sexuality. Couples may wish to continue sexual relations. Because of pain, disability, or previous mutilating surgery such as colostomy or mastectomy, they may find it distasteful or difficult. Frank discussions between partners can help a lot, as can a sympathetic and caring carer by encouraging the couple to discuss their difficulties. There are support groups who provide confidential counselling and advice (Appendix 2).

Many find the more intimate procedures difficult. Generally we are not used to either doing these for others or having others do them for us. A sensitive doctor or nurse will often pick up cues about this and can arrange for a nurse to undertake such tasks or, where it is intolerable for either patient or carer, perhaps the answer is to admit the patient to a hospital or hospice.

A quite normal phenomenon prior to death and which is a potential cause of stress is that of 'anticipatory grief' or what Janis[7] describes as 'the work of worry'. This may occur at any time, especially when the patient is confused or unconscious. It almost seems as if the person the relative knew has ceased to exist and although *si vis vitam, para mortem* (the dying still share life with the living), it is not the person they knew and loved. During this process, the relative tends to have an overwhelming sense of loss, deep sorrow, guilt, anger and depression. They may also explore such issues as 'what will become of me?', 'where shall I live?', 'how shall I manage?' This type of grief may be perceived as unfeeling and uncaring, engendering tension and stress. If they are reassured that this is normal and that it is perfectly in order to grieve in this way, then this can be most helpful.

Encouraging patients and relatives to talk to each other is always extremely beneficial. Often they need 'permission' to talk about the good times they have shared, their disappointments, their hopes and their fears. Such communication can help to allay anxieties on both sides and make this final phase of the patient's life rich and rewarding for him/her and the family. Putting them in touch with a support group may be helpful, particularly in the case of a dying child. Useful addresses, such as that for the Compassionate Friends, may be found in Appendix 2.

Many people procrastinate about such things as making a will. Relatives may be reluctant to discuss such matters for fear of causing distress. If such matters are dealt with, the patient is provided with the chance to clarify his or her wishes after death. The carer is helped in the post-bereavement phase by knowing that they are carrying out these wishes. The family solicitor may be brought in to take care of such matters, though this must obviously be with the consent of the patient. The family's minister of religion, who may be well-known to the patient, can give much support during this difficult time. For the patient, he can provide spiritual consolation and administer sacraments where appropriate.

If the patient needs to be admitted to a hospital or hospice the family may feel a sense of guilt or failure that they were unable to cope until the end. When a patient is admitted everyone should be made to feel welcome. If possible a nurse should meet the ambulance to greet the patient and the family members, who should always be addressed by name so that they retain their dignity and know they are expected. The nurse should try to discuss any special information that the carer has; after all they are the ones who have been most involved until now. This can be done in a friendly and relaxed way, perhaps over a cup of tea, offering encouragement and praise for the way they have managed at home. The admitting nurse should give relatives information about such things as visiting times, telephone numbers, routines and what to bring in for the patient. Often it is helpful if these are written down, since the relative may be distressed. Many hospitals have small booklets containing such useful informaton which provides a good source of reference. Assure the family that their loved one is in safe, secure and caring hands. Introduce the members of the team by name and, if appropriate, explain the different uniforms. Encourage the relatives to participate in the care if they wish. Some relatives feel duty bound to visit at each and every visiting time, for many this is difficult and will compound their tiredness. They may welcome the suggestion that they need a rest and if they are assured that the patient is in capable hands, may feel less guilty about taking it. If it is appropriate, arrangements may be made for the relatives to stay in the hospital or hospice, in any event they should be made to feel welcome.

One of the stresses encountered is the lack of privacy. It is sometimes impossible to have intimate conversations in a busy hospital ward, even behind closed curtains. In one instance in a busy ward, one leukaemic patient and his wife used to disappear to the bathroom each afternoon because it was the one place they could be assured privacy! Some hospices have family rooms which no-one is permitted to enter without knocking.

As the patient's condition deteriorates, the family need information about what to expect. Simple explanations about such things as changes in the patient's colour can help. One of the things which can cause much distress is the 'death rattle'. This, as has been seen, can be ameliorated by drugs, but if a simple explanation is given that it is merely a collection of secretions at the back of the throat, then this can be most reassuring.

In the final stages of the patient's illness the relatives may wish to stay by the bedside and may find it supportive to have a nurse or minister of religion present. When the death occurs they may wish to stay with the deceased for a while. Following this they should be taken to a quiet room and if they wish, the doctor should be available to see them. Encourage them to talk and to cry if they wish. It is a good idea to ask them to return the next day for the certificate and belongings.

When they collect the death certificate they need information as to how and where to register the death and how to go about arranging the funeral. The DHSS publish a helpful booklet *What to do After a Death*. It is important that the information about registrars is written down since the relative is distressed and likely to forget. Most hospitals and hospices provide their own information sheet.

Registration of death and arranging the funeral are distressing times for the family and it may be helpful to have someone accompany them. A sympathetic funeral director can be a great help and many of them have had bereavement training. Bereavement itself is, of course, stressful and this will be dealt with in detail in Chapter 15.

Professional carers

Everyone is aware that any type of work has a potential to be stressful, indeed many millions of working days are lost annually in the UK from short-term absences due to stress. It is estimated that this drains the Exchequer of some £55 million annually in national insurance and social security benefits alone (1989 figures). Palliative care team members are therefore not alone in their stress, although it is becoming increasingly recognized as being a hazard for those in the caring professions. Indeed it has been suggested that caring should carry a government health warning!

Why are the members of caring professions subject to so much stress? Firstly it must be remembered that each member of the team is a human being, reacting and feeling like everyone else. Often, however, they are expected to remain detached, objective and emotionally uninvolved. Even the professional carer can, at times, feel helpless.

The stress may result from their own life styles, from the work itself or from the work organization. Since it is not always possible to avoid the stresses of work, it is clearly important to cope with stress in our individual lives. So, we must try to identify those things which cause us stress, changing those things which we can and learning to cope more effectively with those we cannot. Everyone, especially those involved in palliative care, needs to develop a personal philosophy of life, death and dying which will help sustain them. Everyone needs to relax, take adequate rest and have a healthy diet. Often it is difficult to turn off at the end of a spell of duty. Perhaps it is helpful to learn to unwind on the way home from work; to concentrate on something positive and pleasant rather than on the negative happenings which may have beset us during the day. This is useful in that it helps to separate work and home life.

Many people find exercise a good way to relax. This may take the form of a walk or a more strenuous type of activity such as squash, competitive sports, however, also carry with them the potential for stress. Some may find yoga or meditation helpful, listening to music, reading or hobbies which provide change and relief from the stresses of the day. No doubt each one will have a pet 'unwind' mechanism. It is important to pursue these and to fit into each day a little time for ourselves. This is sometimes difficult to achieve but is an absolute necessity if we are to retain our own well-being. Above all, it is necessary to retain the ability to laugh and play.

Individuals who work in the caring field are often highly motivated to help others. This can lead to them being 'used' outside work by friends, neighbours or relatives. Sometimes it is necessary for them to say 'no' to such calls, otherwise they end up drained emotionally and physically with the sense of never being off duty.

Palliative care encompasses emotional commitment as well as both physical and cognitive ability. It is difficult at times not to get emotionally involved with the patients and their families, particularly if the team cares or supports them over a long period of time. The carer may be hurt and grieved when the patient dies; they too have the need to grieve and mourn at times, it is part of humanity. Multiple deaths obviously create much stress and the team need time to recover. The system needs to have built into it some mechanism whereby this can happen, otherwise morale is seriously affected and individuals become tired, dispirited and there is the potential for 'burn-out'. Some hospices have formal support groups for their staff which may go some way towards ameliorating stress. Often, however, it is the more informal peer group which helps most.

When caring for young people who are dying, when a family is about to lose a child, or a parent is about to die leaving a young family, the problem of the carer identifying with the patient's circumstances may arise. General practitioners may experience this, particularly where they have known a patient really well, perhaps even from birth. No-one is immune. It is not easy to distance oneself but somehow we have to learn to deal with the inherent stress. Perhaps by talking things over with a sympathetic counsellor we may come to see that we have played our part and done our best to help to ameliorate any of the difficulties for the patient, and this may lessen some of the stress. Each one, no doubt, has to develop some sort of coping mechanism in such situations.

Communication may represent a problem for some carers, particularly when dealing with bereaved relatives. Many are afraid of saying the wrong thing. Here education can help by allowing the individuals to explore the nature of verbal and non-verbal communciation and breaking bad news. It is helpful to know that since we are dealing with individuals, there is no *one* right way to deal with such situations. As long as the facts are presented truthfully, sympathetically and in a positive manner which may readily be understood, neither the relatives nor the patient will expect more. Some difficulties may arise in communicating with patients and relatives from different cultural or ethnic backgrounds. Language may present a barrier but lists of interpreters are available. Most courses concerning preparation for palliative care explore aspects of communication with, and the needs of, such people.

Dealing with angry patients and relatives is always difficult but if we are aware of what is happening, that the anger is not necessarily aimed at the carer or the family but is merely a manifestation of frustration, a normal emotional reaction, then we are better able to cope. Education can help us to appreciate what is happening and we are thus less likely to react adversely or to take it personally. We can also help the relatives understand that this is a perfectly normal response and may be able to forestall other potentially distressing situations.

Lack of knowledge is a real stressor. Until recently, both medical and nurse training paid little attention to how one deals with death and dying. The emphasis was largely on the curative aspects of care. Thus death came to be regarded as a failure. Gradually this situation has changed and more recently greater emphasis is being given to the topic in curricula. However, it should also be remembered that each of us has a responsibility for our own knowledge and should thus strive to keep ourselves up-to-date.

Work load is another important consideration. If an individual perceives that there is too much to do this may lead to anxiety and panic, and/or overload, which in itself is a potent cause of stress. Of course, too little work can also be stressful. The team leader needs to monitor what is happening and should endeavour to see that there is equity in the distribution of work.

Communication within the team itself and between the team and other agencies, may represent a potential for stress. This may occur if the team members do not know each other well and are unaware of each other's abilities and expertise. The converse may be true, when the team members know each other too well and not only work together but also socialise together. This can lead to insularity and few outside interests, causing tiredness, anxiety and inability to escape from the job. Clearly, the latter is unsatisfactory and we all need to be able to get away. Good orientation and induction programmes may ameliorate initial difficulties by introducing individuals to the philosophy and objectives of the caring organization. Such programmes introduce role relationships, and provide an opportunity to meet and get to know the other team members. Lack of cohesion may occur within the team itself, this may be due to a rapid turnover of staff preventing them from knowing each other well. This may lead to feelings of vulnerability and provides little potential for development of good peer support systems which are the bedrock for individuals coping with stress. Where there is rapid turnover of staff the cause needs to be explored. It may be that one reaction to too much stress is to leave.

All of us from time to time need positive reinforcement or encouragement to maintain our motivation. Managers and team leaders need to be aware of this, it is all too easy to give negative feedback, picking out those things which have been badly handled, and forgetting the good things. In some instances, for example with Macmillan Nurses, who are not working from a hospital or hospice, there may be feelings of working in isolation or quite simply loneliness. Effective communication systems can go a long way to assuage this. Links can be forged with others working in the speciality, leading to formation of support groups.

In conclusion then, palliative care carries with it great potential for stress both for the patient's relatives and for the professional carers. For the relatives this may be eased by support from the team, good communication, respite care and the knowledge that their loved one is well cared for. For the professional carers the job itself, the individuals own life style and the organization in which they work can be potential sources of stress. Effective life style management, education, good inter- and intra-team communication and caring management may help to reduce some of the stresses.

References

1 Selye, H. (1974) *Stress without Distress*. The New American Library, New York.
2 Lazarus, R. (1966) *Psychological Stress and the Coping Process.* McGraw−Hill, New York.

3 McGrath, J.E. (1970) A conceptual formulation for research on stress. In J.E. McGrath (Ed.) *Social and Psychological Factors in Stress*. Holt, Rinehart & Winston, New York.
4 Jacobson, S. (1985) The context of nurses' stress. In S. Jacobson (Ed.) *Nurses Under Stress*. Wiley, New York.
5 Bailey, R.D. (1985) *Coping with Stress in Caring*. Blackwell Scientific Publications, Oxford.
6 Gaye, J.E. (1986) Nursing under stress. *Journal of Occupational Health* **0**:179−183.
7 Janis, I.L. (1958) *Psychological Stress*. Wiley, New York.

14 The hospice and education for palliative care

The word hospice derives from the Latin *hospitium*, a stranger or guest. From this stem a number of words such as host, hospitable, hospital and hospice. Originally a hospice was a place of entertainment for strangers where a host (one who entertains strangers) would be hospitable (kind to strangers). Sometimes, though archaically, the word hospice is used synonymously for pub. Considering the affection which most British people have for the national institution of the pub this is perhaps the happiest association. In rural parts of England pubs were often built to house stone masons working on building parish churches and in a few cases they even belong to the parish and their proceeds contributed to the vicar's stipend. So pubs too sometimes have a religious aspect. Originally the word hospital had nothing to do with the sick but was a place for receiving pilgrims or a charitable institution for the elderly, infirm or orphaned. In the latter case it may have had an educational role as, for example, in the public school, Christ's Hospital, which was originally founded in 1552 as an orphanage. So the word hospice is deeply trenched in concepts of receiving strangers and cherishing them kindly with sustenance, entertainment and with education.

History

The history of the hospice movement could be said to have started in the middle ages with charitable monastic institutions set up by religious orders. More realistically it can be dated form the foundation of St Luke's Hospital for the Incurable in London in 1893. St Luke's was followed by St Joseph's Hospice in the East End of London in 1905. So the hospice concept was established before the work of Dame Cicely Saunders and the foundation of St Christopher's Hospice in 1967. But it was she who, by establishing high standards of care and thoroughness of research, began to make the subject of palliative care medically as well as socially and humanitarianly respectable. Dame Cicely attributes the concept of St Christopher's to a single Polish patient, David Tasma, whom she met on her first ward as a social worker in St Thomas's Hospital in 1947. She had to tell him about his diagnosis and the way in which together they coped with that news led to the foundation of St Christopher's Hospice[1].

Now in 1989 there are 93 independently managed hospices with a total of 2349 beds.[2]. There are an additional 31 NHS units with 476 beds and several more will open before the end of the year. In addition, there are 231 teams offering palliative care skills within the patients' own homes and a further

21 teams providing advisory services within hospitals. In November 1987, the Royal College of Physicians recognized palliative medicine as a new sub-speciality of general medicine and approved a formal training programme for future consultants in the sub-speciality. This programme allows for senior registrar posts to be set up in approved hospices. Among the prerequisites for such a senior registrarship will be membership of the Royal Colleges including that of the General Practitioners. This means that general practitioners may become consultants in palliative medicine after many years experience of practice.

Modern palliative medicine has much strength but some weakness. It still carries with it an air of 'do-goodery'; a certain piety not born of religion but more of self-satisfaction by its practitioners in both medicine and nursing which puts it at variance with the cultivated objectivity of scientific professionalism. For this reason some people object to the term 'Hospice Movement' which smacks of evangelicism with more than a hint that other practitioners are not 'saved'. This presents a real attitudinal barrier to the extension of the knowledge, skills and attitudes which constitutes the discipline of palliative medicine. This attitudinal barrier, combined with widespread misconceptions of the role and function of hospices and frank ignorance of modern methods of pain control presents a major challenge to the new discipline and its teaching.

A review in the Lancet[3] drew attention to a need for co-ordination in planning and provision of terminal care services which does not alway fit with local enthusiasms. There is a need to harness idealism since the days of uncontrolled growth of hospices are over and there has been little impartial review of hospice performance on a large scale. Parkes has compared hospice and hospital terminal care[4,5] and Wilkes [6] has shown that the quality of care in the patient's own home is very variable. What is needed is a global view of the need for symptom control in the community so that the success or failure of measures designed to meet that need may be measured. A start can be made by reviewing the function of individual hospices and comparing this with their objectives.

Table 14.1 shows a picture of a single small hospice's annual workload which may help to correct misconceptions about its function. Two thirds of its referrals come from general practitioners, another tenth from primary care nurses and about a fifth from hospitals. Most of these referrals are looked after by the primary care teams based on general practices. The hospice home care team support the primary care team with assistance from their medical director who will visit the patients at the request of the general practitioner or the home care sister with the general practitioner's approval. Many patients attend the day care centre where they have the opportunity to discuss their progress with medical and nursing staff and, perhaps more important still, with each other. The day centre provides peer group support, recreational and social functions and facilities for dressings, checking medication, bathing and hairdressing. It often comes as a surprise to people with little experience of hospices that two-fifths of admissions are discharged home alive. About equal numbers of patients die at home as in the hospice and a further fifth die in hospital. Of course there are a large number of deaths, but many patients attend the hospice for periods measured in years. For these people especially the hospice is about living, not about dying.

Table 14.1.   Referrals and workload St Giles Hospice, Lichfield − 1 April 1986 to 31 March 1987

REFERRALS

Source of referral	Staffs	Warwicks	Derby	Leics	N.B'ham	Walsall	Total	(%)
GP	234	19	2	2	32	20	309	(64.1)
Hospital	62	14	3	0	18	5	102	(21.2)
District nurse	42	1	0	0	3	0	46	(9.5)
Social worker	2	0	0	0	0	0	2	(0.4)
Patient	0	0	0	0	1	0	1	(0.2)
Relative of patient	2	0	0	0	1	0	3	(0.6)
Walsall home Care Team	2	0	0	0	0	17	19	(4.0)
Total	344	34	5	2	55	42	482	(100)
%	71.3	7.0	1.0	0.4	11.4	8.7		

TOTAL WORKLOAD

New referrals	482
Patients cared for by home care team:	
Mean no. of per month	155
Range	129−193
Total visits by home care team	2193
Admissions to St Giles: new	196
re-admissions	61
total	257
Live discharges	105 (40.8%)
Total deaths (some patients from 1985−6)	396
of which in hospice	147 (37.1%)
at home	174 (43.9%)
in hospital	75 (19.0%)
Attending day centre	126
Total attendances at day centre	1324

Relationship with general practice

The attitude of many general practitioners was summarized by Akerman in a letter to the British Medical Journal in 1984:

'Like most general practitioners I believe that care of the dying is very much part of our job and we should look to the hospice to help us to do this better − not to do it for us'[7]

There is a generally held view that the best place to die is in one's own bed in one's own home. This is not always possible for many reasons. Chief among these is the lack of suitable support at home and this is becoming an increasing problem with the aging of the population. Another factor lies in relationships between hospices and some primary care teams, where, unfortunately there is evidence of strain. This must reflect on patient care and it is impossible to teach effectively where relations are strained. Standards still vary enormously in general practice, and although an increasing number of first class, well equipped and motivated practices offer excellent care to terminally ill patients in their own homes this is by no means universal. Poor quality of practice creates a bad view of the capabilities of general practitioners, which may well account for the poor opinion that hospice staff sometimes have of them. Such criticism, sensed by good and poor general practitioners alike, tends to increase the distance between primary care teams and the hospice.

In an attempt to explore this anecdotal evidence, that relationships between general practitioners and hospices are strained, a questionnaire was sent to all heads of departments of general practice listed as members of the Association of University Teachers of General Practice. Though academic general practitioners do not represent general practice as a whole, they are an important and influential part of it. Each academic was asked about relations between hospices and general practice in his or her part of Britain, whether they were improving or deteriorating, for an indication of problem areas and how relations might be improved.

Twenty-eight departments responded; some departmental heads deputing the task of replying to colleagues who themselves worked in hospices. The response yielded much detailed information which is summarised in Table 14.2.

Table 14.2 Response to questionnaires about relationships between academic GPs and hospices.

Relationships		Change		Problem areas		Possible solutions	
Excellent	2	Improving	6	Nursing	7	Improve teaching	7
Good	5	Deteriorating	6	Medical	5	Personal contact	6
Fair	16					More GP involvement in hospice	6
Poor	3					More GP/spec. care of patients	2
No comment	2					Change in religious attitudes	1
						No comment	8

The finding that only a quarter of departments consider relationships to be good or excellent, and some to even be deteriorating, is disquieting. Problems occurred with Macmillan nurses in home care teams, and medical staff were criticized about rigidity of admission criteria. There was a fear that the trend for hospices to take over from general practitioners would result in a de-skilling of staff and subsequent deterioration in care standards.

More teaching and involvement of general practitioners in hospices were seen as solutions. Five respondents said relations were better where medical directors were general practitioners, though this did not mean that all GP medical directors enjoyed good relations, or that medical directors from other disciplines suffered bad relations, with their academic department. These findings reflect tensions existing between sources of care. Improvement in palliative care can only come through education and there is a need to measure and define strain between carers before teaching can be successful.

A few verbatim comments from academic general practice are illuminating:

A few Macmillan nurses adopted a condescending attitude to a few socially isolated GPs.

There was initial suspicion by GPs of Macmillan nurses by doctors sensitive about their caring role in a highly emotional area of practice.

Relations indifferent to begin with but improved following 'forthright discussion' . . . relationships that were bad have got better.

My gut feeling about the poor relationship that appears to exist between some hospices and GPs is because GPs are wary at yet another speciality taking patients away from their care.

The de-skilling specialist model is the reason for what I would see as the possibly deteriorating relationships between hospices and GPs . . . there is the same rather uneasy relationship between Macmillan nurses and district nurses as exists between palliative care specialists and GPs.

Lest these views sound nihilistic a quarter of replies found that relationships were good or excellent and several departmental heads commented that they respected the work of Cancer Relief and were keen to work towards a constructive outcome for all concerned.

Table 14.2 reveals that while in many areas the situation is improving, six heads of GP departments believe it to be getting worse. So here is clear evidence of a problem. Haines and Booroff[8], in a study of London general practice, found that half of the GPs felt that they needed more training in symptom control and 40% said they needed training in communication. The conclusion is obvious: basic education is inadequate and this is true of all who care for cancer patients: doctors, nurses, social workers and clergy.

One must be concerned at the way in which general practice and palliative care which, in co-operation, have so much to offer very sick people are in danger of conflict. Such conflict must diminish patient care. So it behoves all who work in palliative care to analyse the difficulties which exist and to bridge them rather than assuming adversarial and competitive positions. It is all too easy to respond to criticism with anger or self-justification which achieves nothing.

The solution to these problems lies, as it always does in relationship difficulties, in improved communication. One way that this might be achieved is through the use of a co-operation card, in the way that general practitioners and obstetricians do for shared antenatal care. This possibility is being explored in a multidisciplinary committee at the Queen Elizabeth Hospital, Birmingham (see p. 138). But what is really needed is to get people to talk and listen to each other. That is easily said, but far less easily accomplished because it is so difficult to get the people concerned into a situation where they can talk and listen. In the undergraduate field it is comparatively easy and the recent establishment of academic posts in palliative care in several medical schools must help this. But, while improved undergraduate teaching is good, it takes many years to show effect.

A report of a survey funded by a Royal College of General Practitioners Schering scholarship in 1987[9] of vocational training courses showed a deficiency in palliative care teaching: 17% of 172 training schemes devote less than 2% of curriculum time to terminal care and bereavement, 57% spend between 2 and 6% and only 5% spend 10% or more on these subjects, which are so important in the establishment of the doctor–patient relationship. Vocational training is an area where a huge amount of educational effort is made and it is sad that there should be so little teaching on the care of patients with advanced cancer and their relatives.

Hospice facilities should be used to encourage postgraduate education aimed at both primary and secondary care. This should not just be in palliative care but in broad aspects of medicine as a whole and particularly about AIDS. From this broad base it should be possible to introduce the teaching of symptom control and communication skills.

References

1 Saunders, C. (Ed.) (1981) *Hospice: the Living Idea.* Edward Arnold, London.
2 Hillier, R. (1988) Palliative medicine; a new speciality. *British Medical Journal* **297**:874–875.
3 Editorial (1986) Hospice comes of age. *Lancet* **1**:1013–1014.
4 Parkes, C.M. (1978) Home or hospital? Terminal care as seen by surviving spouses. *Journal of the Royal College of General Practitioners* **12**:19–22.
5 Parkes, C.M. & Parkes, J. (1984) 'Hospice' versus 'hospital' care— re-evaluation after ten years as seen by surviving spouses. *Postgraduate Medical Journal* **601**:120–124.
6 Wilkes, E. (1984) Dying now. *Lancet* **1**:950–952.

7 Akerman, F. (1984) Hospices (correspondence). *British Medical Journal* **288**:1996.

8 Haines, A. & Booroff, A. (1986) Terminal care at home: perspectives from general practice. *British Medical Journal* **292**: 1051 − 1053.

9 Richards, C.M. (1987) *The Teaching of Terminal Care and Care of the Bereaved in VTS Schemes.* RCGP Schering Scholarship Report, London.

15 Terminal care and bereavement

Terminal care

When palliative care has been conducted well the emphasis of care, right at the end, may shift from the patient to the family. The strain of caring for a close relative at home is enormous. Such strain can be borne more easily where relatives feel themselves members of the nursing and medical team and it is important to tell them how well they are doing. Sometimes when it all over-whelms the relative a few words of encouragement and praise from a respected doctor or nurse can give new heart. Those who have looked after their dying children, spouse or parent may feel glad at having done so and their subsequent bereavement may be easier. For the doctor there can be few tasks so satisfying as well-conducted care of a family through such a death.

The change from palliative care to terminal care is not easy to define since both are concerned with the quality of the patient's life. There comes a point, however, when further active treatment designed to improve quality of life may actually diminish it. Here one comes into difficult transitional areas since some may argue that to withhold treatment that could prolong life is tantamount to euthanasia (Appendix 3). Euthanasia is a much misused word which really means 'good death' (Greek: *eu*, good; *thanatos*, death), 'a consummation devoutly to be wished'. But euthanasia has come to mean 'assisted death'. There is an artificial division of such action into active (i.e. deliberate killing) and passive euthanasia (the withholding of a drug or procedure which might prolong life but which in the opinion of the carer would unbearably reduce the quality of life). The former, in our opinion, is unacceptable, the latter humane. There comes a time when, in the presence of terminal infection, haemorrhage, con-fusion, convulsions, respiratory failure or profound metabolic disturbance, treatment should be aimed at improving the quality of what life remains rather than merely prolonging it. A good rule is to ask oneself whether the proposed treatment would distress the patient more than the symptoms it aims to ameliorate. In such a decision the views of relatives and the whole team should be considered.

Respiratory problems

Terminal pneumonia, often referred to in the past as 'the old man's friend', rarely responds to antibiotics and their prescripton serves only to prolong the agony for relatives. The difficulty comes in deciding when such pneumonia is in fact terminal rather than an intercurrent episode in what may, thanks to excellent palliative care, be a long period of good quality life.

A late symptom which is very distressing to relatives and, in hospitals or hospices, perhaps to other patients, is the noisy terminal respiration of the dying. The tachypnoea that often occurs may be slowed with intravenous diamorphine and the noise (the death rattle) may be eased and quietened with hyoscine.

Very rarely there may be mediastinal haemorrhage sufficient to cause acute tracheal obstruction when death may be almost immediate; where there is acute distress, Diazepam should be administered intravenously.

Other problems

Terminal confusion can be extremely distressing to exhausted relatives since it appears that the patient is suffering. When additional sedation is necessary methotrimeprazine by syringe driver will ensure a more peaceful end. Similarly, severe convulsions due to cerebral lesions or to uraemia will require sedation, usually via syringe driver, when opioids and methotrimeprazine may be more satisfactory than conventional anticonvulsants.

Serious bleeding is fortunately very rare but when it occurs is very frightening to the patient, relatives or other patients. It may occur due to rupture of a large vessel into a main bronchus, the stomach, rectum or vagina. When the bleeding is arterial, death is often rapid but in the commoner venous bleeding it may be slow and terrifying. Intravenous sedation is required with Diazepam and/or diamorphine. The quantity of blood lost can be very frightening and the use of red towels will help to minimise distress. Following such an event there will be a need for support by all the medical and nursing staff involved. Relatives witnessing such a death may require long-term counselling.

Severe hypercalcaemia is another condition in which it may be appropriate to treat the patient symptomatically since intravenous lines, frequent venesection and the administration of drugs such as mithramycin may be intolerable for the patient.

Bereavement

Bereavement is normally associated with the death of a close relative, friend or even a much loved pet, but in fact occurs in any state of loss.

Though death is probably the commonest cause of bereavement it may also occur after material loss such as a stock market crash or following a broken love affair. The term 'broken heart' has been used since time immemorial to describe the pain of the end of a romance and individuals undergoing such heartbreak follow exactly the same process as those bereft by death. In addition the term heartbreak may literally be true, because those suffering from bereavement are more prone to serious physical disease such as infection, cancer and heart attack than similar groups of non-bereaved people.

Stages of bereavement

Elisabeth Kübler-Ross[1] in her seminal book, *Death and Dying*, describes stages of the bereavement reaction as follows:
1 Denial, isolation and searching.
2 Anger.
3 Depression.
4 Acceptance.

It is important to realise that patients with advanced cancer are themselves undergoing bereavement in that they too are shortly to be deprived of life, their loved ones and all their treasured possessions. They too go through the same stages in the process of coming to terms with impending death but here Kübler-Ross adds the additional stage of bargaining as a third stage between those of anger and depression. Though these stages can be clearly distinguished they may run together or overlap and are rarely as clear cut as the original Kübler-Ross classification would suggest. Though there may be considerable variations with culture, some form of grief reaction is ubiquitous.

Denial, isolation and searching

In the first stage, especially where death has been very sudden, there is often total disbelief of the news when it is given. Those who have the awful job of breaking news of sudden death may be astonished at first reactions which sometimes appear heartless in their non-acceptance. This non-belief is at first because the bereaved person cannot accept, and later will not accept, the bad news. Later still, when acceptance of the news as fact seems to have ocurred there may be a return to non-belief, this time as denial of what is really known, but whose admission is temporarily impossible. Again, one sees this frequently in dying patients, who may have been talking earlier and quite matter-of-factly about death and who later choose to pretend that they are unaware of its approach. Both the bereaved and the dying may try to isolate themselves as part of their denial so that others may not bring them back to the reality they shun. Another aspect of this stage of grieving is searching, when the bereaved person seeks the dead in all those places where he or she might have been found before. At this time there is a tendency to mistake others for the lost person who may be mistakenly seen in crowds or walking in the street. Sometimes the conviction of seeing the dead person is so strong that the bereaved person will run after people and accost them. The following experience of one of us (RH) illustrates this.

As a student I had been climbing in Snowdonia and was hitchhiking back to London, I had been away several days and was in climbing clothes with a rucksack, boots, ice axe and rope. Night was falling and I had almost abandoned getting a lift when a car stopped and an elderly Welshman got out with two younger men. The older man wanted to know who I was and where I was going. The younger men seemed very angry at something. It transpired that they had just driven from Lancaster where they had been to identify the body of the old man's son and younger mens' brother who had been killed while hitchhiking from a climbing holiday in the Lake District. He was my age, dressed as I was, had a few days beard and he too had had a rucksack with boots, rope and ice axe. In the fading light, the father was convinced that I was his son. To the undisguised annoyance of the brothers the father insisted on driving me some hundred miles, stopping to buy drinks and a meal. When they finally put me down the old Welshman got out of the car and, with tears streaming down his face, kissed me goodbye. As a 22-year-old student, I found that difficult to cope with; perhaps I inadvertently gave some solace to that grieving father, he certainly taught me a great deal about bereavement.

Anger

Anger is a common reaction to bad news, whether it be about prognosis or the news of death. Among cancer patients anger is frequently directed at the carer. Sometimes this is displacement, as the patient is really angry at God for having abandoned or cursed him or her with cancer. Sometimes the carer may, justifiably or otherwise, appear to be culpable. We all have to learn to accept that being recipients for the anger of grief is part of our role and that its acceptance is far more helpful to the bereaved than its rejection. It is not always easy to respond in this fashion but the turning of the cheek is more effective in dealing with this sort of anger than any other. Anger may be turned on the person who has died: 'Why did he go and leave me?' One of our patients whose much-loved husband took her out for dinner and suffered a fatal myocardial infarct between entree and dessert told us angrily afterwards 'and the silly beggar didn't even pay the bill!' Anger may take the form of guilt and rage at self: 'Why didn't I . . . '. Guilt is an extremely common component of bereavement and frequently those left behind will want to go over every detail of the dead person's last days, seeking times and places where they could have done more and blaming themselves irrationally for tiny details.

Depression

Gradually anger fades to be replaced by apathy and depression. Here depression is usually reactive and eventually recovers but should be observed for signs suggesting its deepening into severe potentially suicidal endogenous depression (see Chapter 9). In dying patients, a different phase of bargaining may become apparent at this stage. It takes the form of offering to trade with fate or God. 'If you take this away or make it a bad dream then I will . . . ' and all sorts of bargains may be offered. It is sad that enormous energy and resource may be put into this exercise, and patients may exhaust themselves dragging round the country to leave no stone unturned in their effort to strike bargains of cure. This may involve religious pilgrimage, or seeking extravagant claims of cure as a means of clutching at straws. Persuading the patient to take rational decisions in the face of bargaining is very difficult.

Acceptance

Ultimately the bereaved come to accept their loss and resume a normal but different life. Sometimes acceptance itself is a cause of guilt, 'How can I live a normal life without him?' Sometimes renewal of sexual interest seems betrayal of the dead and may require very delicate counselling. Anniversaries may be a time of recurrence of bereavement for years after loss. Many general practitioners will be aware of clustering of consultations round a given date over several years and the question 'Did anything ever happen to you about this time of year?' may well unleash the catharsis of tears.

Pattern of bereavement

The pattern of normal grief is well-illustrated in the diagram from Brown and Stoudemire[2] which shows emotional, somatic, cognitive and motivational effects of grief at phases of initial shock, preoccupation with the deceased and resolution (Fig. 15.1). Normal bereavement runs a variable course, some people recover quickly while others may take a year or more to make a new life. In some respects the nature of the terminal illness may influence this. Where patient and relatives have had time to adjust to the inevitability of death, bereavement is often easier (or may even have been conducted before death) than where it is sudden or unexpected. Where the relatives have had the opportunity to tend the dying individual and to express their love, bereavement may be much easier because of the expiation of real or imagined guilt towards the dying person.

A peculiar but quite common feature of grief is hallucination. This may occur in any bereavement but is commoner between spouses particularly after long and successful marriage.

Occasionally an abnormal bereavement pattern may develop with severe and pathological exaggeration of any of its stages. Denial can lead to a schizoid withdrawal from reality as in Miss Haversham's behaviour, described by Dickens in *Great Expectations* when she developed a denial of reality after the cancellation of her wedding and preserved the wedding feast ever afterwards.

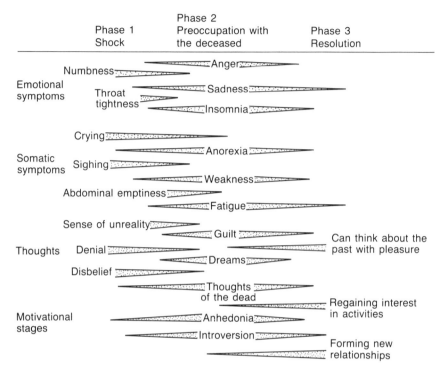

Fig 15.1   Phases of uncomplicated grief.

Anger may be so extreme as to develop into vendetta; but these behaviour patterns are fortunately rare. A much commoner abnormal grief reaction leads to severe depression with classical early morning waking, feelings of worthlessness and loss of future. In such cases suicide is a potential risk. There are a number of risk factors with predictive value for pathological grief which include low social class, male gender and youth. Religious activity and personality show only weak correlations with severe bereavement reactions but the duration and nature (especially violent or suicidal death) of the terminal illness are important indicators of abnormal grief. The state of the marital relationship is also important, especially where the remaining spouse had felt dependent upon or ambivalent towards the dead person. Where pathological bereavement is predicted, intervention may reduce the risk of physical or psychological ill-health through counselling. The encouragement of grief work, in which the grieving individual works through a number of situations which closely involve the dead person, may assist a return to normality.

Morbidity of bereavement

Bereavement has a substantial mortality and morbidity. For centuries it has been observed that death rates are higher among the bereaved than the non-bereaved. Recent work has shown that this effect may be produced as a result of altered catecholamine metabolism in the brain which may lead to altered behaviour patterns and abnormal stress reactions. Altered catecholamine metabolism may have a direct affect on the cardiovascular system leading to raised blood pressure, heart failure and myocardial infarction. But there is also evidence of changes in the immune system, especialy on T-lymphocyte function, in bereavement and allied emotional states (see Chapter 11).

Management

The management of bereavement depends more upon listening than on anything else and as such is very time-consuming. Perhaps this is the reason that it is often neglected, even more so when there is a lingering, nagging doubt in the carer's mind that in fact more *could* have been done. Such doubt is only too human after a death when many aspects of a case may seem regrettable with hindsight. It is good primary care policy to visit all families after a death to ensure that all is well. In the majority of cases it will be, but nothing is lost since the fact that someone appeared to care will be remembered. In those cases where anger or other emotional turmoil smoulder on, a visit may do much to allow ventilation of pent-up feelings. In many cases the carer has no other function than to listen to the chronicle of the deceased's last illness and hours. This is very comforting to those who are left behind who may be able, through talking, to assuage their own conflicting feelings about the death.

It is important to observe the grieving process to ensure that it is not becoming abnormal or that intervention with hypnotics or antidepressants are not necessary. Sometimes this will involve several home visits or attendances at the surgery. Care should be taken to explore particular problems of the bereaved individual. This need not necessarily be done by doctors, often receptionists, nurses, social workers or ministers of religion may be more appropriate. The problem is that with so many who might be involved there is a risk that no-one will be. There is much to be said for a death book (or computerized register) used in primary care to record deaths as they occur. This then allows the practice routine to institute follow-up by the most appropriate carer to check that families are coping. This also provides a source of reference so that anniversaries of deaths may be remembered.

As John Donne reminds us

No man is an island, entire of it self . . . Any man's death diminishes me, because I am involved in Mankind; And therefore never send to know for whom the bell tolls; it tolls for thee.

So one must be aware of the effect of death on a ward, street or locality. For long-stay patients in hospice the frequent experience of death may be very distressing. When, as sometimes happens, there is a cluster of deaths this has its effect upon carers. Occasionally it may be necessary to slow the rate of admissions for a time to allow adjustment, even at the risk of ruining cost-benefit figures. In the community, death may affect a street or neighbourhood. This may lead to patients presenting with concern at the possibility of similar disease as that which killed their friend or neighbour. For example, where a death occurs from breast cancer it is common experience for women who were close to the deceased to be concerned about their own breasts. Wise primary care teams may adapt to this reaction with increased health education. Whole areas may undergo mass grief reactions especially in the presence of multiple deaths or disasters such as the Lockerbie air crash. Such circumstances require the services of specially trained counsellors with experience of disaster care.

References

1   Kübler-Ross, E. (1974) *Death and Dying*. Macmillan, New York.
2   Brown, J.T. & Stoudemire, G.A. (1983) *Journal of the American Medical Association* **250**:378–382.

Further reading

Osterweis, M., Solomon, F. & Green, M. (Eds) (1984) *Bereavement, Reactions, Consequences and Care*. National Academy Press, Washington DC.
Parkes, C.M. (1972) *Bereavement*. Penguin, Harmondsworth.
Stroebe, W. & Stroebe, M.S. (1988) *Bereavement and Health*. Cambridge University Press, Cambridge.

16   Teamwork in palliative care

What is a team?

Most of us have been involved at some time or other in teams, playing football, cricket or hockey or perhaps less athletically in darts, cards or quizzes. These teams all have one thing in common: the solution of a common problem, the attainment of a common goal. Some teams function to achieve an end for all their members some, such as mountaineers, co-operate to put one or two people on top. When Hilary and Tensing reached the summit of Everest this was a team effort crowned by the two individuals. Teamwork in palliative care is more like this than other joint endeavours, in that it aims to succeed primarily for one person: the patient. Of course successful palliative care brings a sense of satisfaction and achievement to all who co-operate, even if, like some of the backup team for Hilary and Tensing they got no further than base camp. But the fact remains that the object of care is the maximization of the patient's quality of life until the end.

Who is in the team?

The members of a team giving palliative care may be many and various. Some of them are listed in Table 1.1 (see p. 2). But this list does not include a number of people who may be in the team; for example, practitioners of complementary therapy (though some allopathic practitioners may be unhappy at their inclusion within the palliative care team). The most glaring omissions, however, are the principal carer, often a close relative or spouse, and the patient him or herself. There is a tendency for some health care workers to exclude the patient from the team seeing him or her as the passive recipient of all the attention rather than being intimately involved in all what is happening; as if Tensing and Hilary were carried bodily to the top of Everest! If you have doubts about this consider your own final illness: would you not want to be involved to some degree in the decision-making about your care and where you might die? This means then that the patient has to be seen as an important member of the team. Once this is accepted then certain implications follow.

Who leads the team?

In the usual caring hierarchy of hospital or general practice the doctor is the leader and principal decision-maker. The decision structure is triangular with instruction passing downwards while information is reported up to the apex of decision, the doctor. In palliative care, when life-saving measures have taken second place to the maximization of quality of life, nurses become more important than doctors for dying patients. It might be more appropriate for the nurse to take over the traditional doctor's role as leader once the decision to palliate rather than cure has been taken. To some doctors this may come as relief since, having been taught to cure, they see no role for themselves once cure has been abandoned; others resent what they see as usurpation of their function. Both these attitudes are disastrous if optimum care is to be provided for the dying patient.

So in palliative care the traditional triangle of leadership has to be abandoned for a circular model in which each professional contributes according to his or her own skills (Fig. 16.1). Where there is need for decision-making this

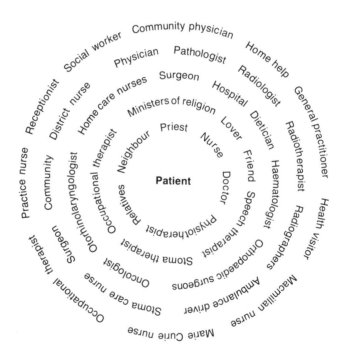

Fig. 16.1   The team in palliative care with the patient at the centre.

should be undertaken by the most appropriate professional (in conjunction with the informed patient) who temporarily may assume the position of *primus inter pares*. Sometimes this leadership may fall on a person without professional responsibility: a neighbour, a friend or most importantly the principal carer be that spouse, parent or child of the patient. The principal carer should always be consulted and frequently encouraged to assume team leadership. It has already been stressed that the patient is the most important person in the team so it follows that at the centre of the circle of carers he or she should also adopt the role of leadership. How often this may occur will depend on the individual personality and the severity of illness.

This adjustment of role demands from all the caring professions a considerable humility; perhaps more than any other quality it is the presence of such humility that separates good carers from bad among those caring for patients with advanced cancer.

Functions of the team

It follows that the function of the team is the optimization of the collective skills of all the members and the willingness to enlist additional skills from outside the team. This again poses some behavioural barriers. The traditional primary care team involving general practitioners, practice and district nurses, the health visitor and perhaps a social worker are used to working together, usually have excellent communication systems and are known to the patient. Sometimes it is difficult for this nuclear team to realize that they may be insufficiently experienced in certain palliative care techniques and deny the patient the expertise of others outside the nuclear team. There may also be interprofessional rivalries or clashes of philosophy or religious beliefs. Though these difficulties should not be overstressed it is only fair to draw attention to them since patients often report them.

From this it will be seen that the first function of a team is to know its own limitations and where additional help may be found. In seeking such help it should be understood by members of the primary care team and those whom they ask for help that the known, trusted faces of the general practitioner and nurse are essential to good palliative care. It is not the function of hospice or any other workers to take over from the general practitioner and nurse, it is their job to support and augment them. There is often still too much possessiveness about caring reflected in the phrase 'my patient'. Such possessiveness may be protective and nobody criticizes a carer who jealously guards his patient against unhelpful interference but the same attitude often militates against the correct use of outside help. This may involve walking a fine line and it is a major function of the team to see that this is done to the best advantage of the patient.

Ethical conflict

Conflict may arise if goals and ethics are not shared by the team members. The decision to adopt palliative care rather than continue aggressive treatment aimed at cure poses difficult decision-making, involving value judgements concerning quantity and quality of life. The whole field of palliative care is filled with ethical questions. Do we prescribe antibiotics for a chest infection? Should we offer a patient a blood transfusion for the relief of today's symptom if it may prolong the agony and make tomorrow's symptom worse? There may be even starker questions where some team members may hold strong and conflicting views. In earlier, more paternalistic days such decisions were sometimes taken by doctors in isolation. That way only one conscience has to be satisfied; it can be much more difficult when several sets of morals have to reach consensus.

Such problems are not uncommon and require recognition and discussion. Where there are questions of the patient's autonomy being threatened by sedation or where admission is arranged for good reason but against the patient's wishes, conflict of opinion may arise as to the wisdom of decision-making leading to real distress within the team. Sometimes a balance has to be struck between a fully alert patient capable of relating to his family and making autonomous decisions and some symptoms such as pain. Sometimes there may be disagreements about the use of opioids near to the end or about the use of steroids or antidepressants such as dexamphetamine. There has to be a mechanism for coping with difficulties which may arise from such problem areas. This requires patient discussion among equals rather than unilateral, dogmatic decisions.

The team and AIDS

In cases of AIDS there are likely to be special difficulties. Experience has shown that real problems posed in the palliative care of AIDS patients are trivial compared with the imagined. The syndrome is surrounded by even more myth and fear than cancer and compounded by all sorts of attitudes built upon prejudice, retributive religious concepts and homophobia. One senior hospice nurse announced that her non-medical professional husband had forbidden her to continue work in the hospice after it admitted its first AIDS patient. With such attitudes, based upon ignorance and fear, in intelligent, informed people what hope is there for the less informed? There is a widespread belief that AIDS patients are highly infective and this frightens some members of the caring professions. Perhaps the relative risks are put in perspective by the following case history.

A young mother had two sons both of whom had haemophilia. The elder boy was HIV + and also developed severe allergy to factor VIII. In consequence he had almost daily bleeds and his mother was always cleaning up his blood. This happened at a very early stage in the development of the AIDS epidemic when she was not aware that there was any risk. Neither she nor her husband took any special precautions while looking after their son. This continued for several years until the boy eventually died from a cerebral haemorrhage. Now, much later, neither of the parents has sero-converted.

In dealing with AIDS the team must be informed and emotionally adjusted to dealing uncritically with people whose sexuality may be different from their own, who are non-judgemental and who respect the human immunodeficiency virus without being terrified of it. Education needs to be channelled directly at multidisciplinary teams. With this aim a group comprising doctors, nurses, social workers and education officers have set up a travelling course which tours the postgraduate centres of the Midlands to increase knowledge and challenge attitudes about AIDS in primary care teams.

The team and complementary medicine

Another area of difficulty already referred to is that of association with non-allopathic practitioners. For a long time this has been taboo, even to the extent of risk of a doctor having his name removed from the medical register. Perhaps under the influence of members of the Royal Family these attitudes are being questioned. There are even glimmerings of scientific explanations for some of the apparently bizarre claims made by practitioners of complementary medicine (see Chapter 11, p. 85). Whatever the truth to such claims the fact that the patient obtains comfort from something that his or her allopathic carers may regard as nonsensical is all important. After all what does palliation do but to give comfort? While cure is possible then the best treatment, as judged by the conventional wisdom of the day, must be right; when cure is impossible then anything which increases the patient's well-being is good and if it boosts the failing immune system at the same time that is good too.

Need for education of the team

All this points to a need for greater education to instil knowledge and skills and, most importantly, to modify attitudes and overcome prejudice. This means educating all the members of the team, including the laity, for they may be carers or patients. The myth and taboo that surrounds cancer militates against good communication within the family of a patient with cancer. Education is needed to break down these barriers which cause so much bitterness, misery and misundertanding. The following case history illustrates one of the common misconceptions about cancer.

> A district nurse reported that whenever she went to bath a man dying of cancer the patient's son always accompanied her to the bathroom where he turned on taps and handed towels. She appreciated this believing that he was very well-mannered but the truth was that he was afraid of catching cancer.

Education of the team requires a combined, interdisciplinary approach involving any and all professions who may be involved in palliative care. Whilst this is easily said it is very difficult to achieve for many reasons. Obviously the physical difficulty of gathering together a number of very busy people is enormous. Though the difference in knowledge between the various team members appears to make it hard to provide education which is not too simple for some and overcomplex for others, it does allow appreciation of each others' skills and roles. A more serious difficulty lies in the fact that those who attend educational meetings are often the best informed and motivated, those most in need stay away.

This need for education is perhaps the most important challenge facing those who work in palliative care and increasingly there is academic representation of the discipline in medical schools. Medical students respond extremely positively to palliative care education and this offers the prospect of better team work in the future. Though it may be difficult to overcome the barriers of curricular and service commitments when groups of nursing, medical and social work students study together there is often a cathartic shake-up of attitudes and assumptions which is healthy, stimulating and fun.

One way of coping with the disparity of knowledge between professional groups is through case discussion, particularly when based on a videotaped case history. Where the videotape is a drama with no attempt at dictating behaviour, attitudes or communication skills the teacher can draw from the group their opinions on what they see and so involve them all in interprofessional discussion. A number of such tapes have been made at Birmingham University.

Importance of communication

In all this communication is most important. There needs to be continuing and easy exchange of information about physical, psychological, social and spiritual aspects of the patient's case. Such information should also involve the patient in so far as he or she wishes. As a means of improving communication throughout the team a scheme called ONCARE (an acronym combining concepts of Ongoing Care with Oncology Care) is being piloted in Birmingham. ONCARE has been devised by a group of professionals working with cancer patients in and around the Queen Elizabeth Hospital. It aims to improve communication between people with cancer and all those who help to care for them. The idea started with the appointment of the Macmillan Senior Lecturer in Palliative Care at the Medical School in Birmingham in 1987. Following this appointment a group of consultants caring for cancer patients asked for suggestions as to how communication could be improved to help their patients. From this initial nucleus the group has grown to include representatives from many branches of medicine, nursing, social work, the clergy and many other caring professions. The group has been discussing the problem and its many attendant difficulties (some of which involved frank professional territorialism) over the past 2 years and has now reached the point where the project can be formally launched.

ONCARE consists of two ideas:

1 The ONCARE card (Fig. 16.2); this is based on an original design by Dr Jim Storer, a general practitioner in Chelmsley Wood, Birmingham, and modified after many committee meetings. It is similar to the co-operation card used in obstetrics which is carried by the patient but allows exchange of information between obstetrician, midwife and general practitioner. In the case of the ONCARE card the patient who wishes to do so will be issued with a card on which notes may be made by any of the patient's carers. ONCARE aims to help patients who wish to have more information about cancer. It also allows sharing of information between all the patient's carers: the family, doctors, nurses, social workers, clergy and anyone else whom the patient may wish to involve. The important aspect of the ONCARE card is that it establishes the patient at the centre of the caring circle and gives him or her custody of information. The patient is thus firmly part of the team and may have as much information as he or she wishes and can ensure that all the carers know what is happening. Of course some peole will not wish such inolvement and that is acceptable. Since the possession, or the reading, of a card will be entirely voluntary those who do not want such information need not join the scheme. The extent to which the individual is involved will be his or her own decision thereby increasing patient autonomy. A prototype of the card has been shown to patients whose response has been very favourable, the vast majority welcoming such an innovation and grateful to have more information about their disease.

2 A meeting place where patients may seek information, such as a coffee shop, where volunteers will listen to problems and steer them towards appropriate sources of advice or counselling. This forum will allow patients who are worried or do not understand their treatment to ask questions or to seek elucidation of entries on the ONCARE card.

ORIGINAL DIAGNOSIS AND SITE | DATE

CURRENT MANAGEMENT
DATE | COMMENTS

for use by doctors, nurses & other carers

| | TEST RESULTS | REVIEW APPT | init |

PLAN (BRIEF STATEMENT OF WHAT YOU HAVE TOLD PATIENT)
DATE

TREATMENT/PROBLEM SUMMARY

0001

SOME POSSIBLE SIDE EFFECTS

you are having treatment for your cancer and its problems. Some times either because of the disease you may experience a variety of symptoms including some of those listed below don't worry about this: some symptoms may be expected at certain stages of treatment and all can be helped by modern medical techniques.

POSSIBLE SIDE EFFECTS	TREATMENT DATES					
Appetite loss						
Bleeding						
Constipation						
Cough						
Diarrhoea						
Discharge						
Dizziness						
Feeling Sick						
Hair change						
Itching						
Pain						
Sex Problems						
Short breath						
Skin changes						
Sleeplessness						
Sore skin						
Vomiting						
Weight change						
Wind						

THE INFORMATION ON THIS CARD MAY HELP YOU, YOUR CARERS AND OTHER PATIENTS

USEFUL INFORMATION

THINGS YOUR DOCTOR WANTS YOU TO REPORT TO HIM URGENTLY (if any)

ARE YOU ENTITLED TO?:-

ATTENDANCE ALLOWANCE
INVALID CARE GRANT
MOBILITY ALLOWANCE
CANCER RELIEF MACMILLAN FUND
HELP FROM DHSS SOCIAL FUND
MALCOLM SARGENT FUND

COULD ANY OF THE FOLLOWING BE USEFUL TO YOU?

SELF HELP GROUP
NAME AND ADDRESS:
HOSPICE:
MACMILLAN NURSE:

ONCARE CARD

During your illness you may meet many Doctors, nurses and other carers. This card will keep you and all your carers informed of what is happening in your case.

PATIENT'S NAME AND ADDRESS | CHANGE OF ADDRESS

TEL: | TEL:
SPECIALIST | HOSPITAL REF. No

TEL: | TEL:
GENERAL PRACTITIONER'S NAME AND ADDRESS (1)

TEL:
GENERAL PRACTITIONER'S NAME AND ADDRESS(2)

TEL:
DISTRICT NURSE NAME AND ADDRESS

TEL:
CARER'S* NAME AND ADDRESS

TEL:

*CARER - Spouse/relative/friend etc

17 Epilogue

Who will care for the majority of cancer patients in the future? Today some 7% of patients with advanced cancer are cared for by hospices and it is unlikely that a much higher proportion will ever benefit directly from hospice care. It follows then that one of the most important roles of hospices is to set an example of care and to educate those primary and secondary care doctors and nurses who will provide palliative care in the community and in district general hospitals.

Throughout this book the term palliative care has been applied almost exclusively to cancer but of course it applies to all other forms of chronic disease as well. The concept of applying the principles of palliative medicine to neurological, rheumatological, even to chronic psychiatric disease implies huge changes in thinking about priorities in medicine and resource allocation. It also requires adoption of new attitudes by all the caring professions especially those of medicine and nursing.[1] With an ever ageing population and people living longer and more productive lives with chronic disease, a change in professional priority from cure to care, from intervention to prevention and rehabilitation, becomes not only desirable but economic. If this is to be achieved then hospices have much to do in leading the way. In the words of an American physician:

> If we are to be successful in having hospice concepts applied to medical areas beyond the terminally ill, we will have to find a better way to reach our colleagues. We ought to stop berating them for being insensitive, lacking in humanity, and for running away from emotions. Our job is to find a more convincing way of reaching them.[2]

In earlier days a doctor's reputation depended on his skills at the birthbed and deathbed. Now that primary care obstetrics is so rare the team must depend upon care of the dying for building up the trust which is so vital between carers and patients. Such care begins at first diagnosis, possibly even before that, and it depends more than anything else upon mutual trust. Good care increases that trust not only with the family of the sick individual but with the wider circle of the patient's extended family and friends, and each such case increases this community trust. This trust confers upon the members of the team a power with which they may influence behaviour such as giving up smoking, changing drinking or sexual behviour.

So one comes full circle: good palliative care of one patient increases the power of the team to prevent disease in others.

References

1 Hull, F.M. (1987) The role of socio-behavioral scientists in health care practice. *Social Science and Medicine* **25**:679–687.
2 Klagsbrun, S.C. (1981) Hospice—a developing role. In C. Saunders (Ed.) *Hospice: the Living Idea*, pp. 5–8. Edward Arnold, London.

Appendix 1: Drugs

This drug list is designed for ready reference only, detailed information on drugs should be sought in the *British National Formulary*. Drugs are listed under symptom headings.

Generic name	Proprietary name	Route of administration	Dose range	Page no.
AIDS				96−106
Amphotericin	Fungilin	Oral	100−200 mg four times daily	103
		i.v.	250 μg/kg/day	
Clindamycin	Dalacin C	Oral	500 mg four times daily	104
Codeine phosphate		Oral	10−60 mg 4-hourly	103
Co-trimoxazole	Septrin	i.v.	20 mg/kg/day	102
Ketoconazole	Nizoral	Oral	200−400 mg daily	103
Loperamide	Imodium	Oral	6−16 mg daily	103
Nystatin	Nystan	Oral	up to 0.5 units four times daily	
Pentamidine		i.v.	2−4 mg/kg/day	102,104
Pyrimethamine	Daraprim	Oral	25 mg daily	103
Zidovudine	Retrovir	Oral	200−300 mg 4-hourly	105
Anorexia				54−55
Alcohol				55
Dexamethasone	Decadron	Oral/s.c.	2−16 mg/day	55
Confusion				61−62
Clormethiazole	Heminevrin	Oral	4−6×250 mg/day	62
Dexamethasone	Decadron	Oral/s.c.	2−16 mg/day	62
Haloperidol	Haldol	Oral/s.c.	1−30 mg/day	62
Methotrimeprazine	Nozinan	s.c.	25−200 mg/day	62
Thioridazine	Melleril	Oral	100−600 mg/day	62
Constipation				51−52
Bulk formers				
Ispaghula	Fybogel	Oral	1−4 sachet/day	52
Methylcellulose	Celevac	Oral	3−6 tabs/day	52
Sterculia	Normacol	Oral	1−4 sachet/day	52
Faecal softeners				
Arachis oil		Enema		
Liquid paraffin		Oral	10−30 ml/day	52
Osmotic laxatives				
Lactulose	Duphalac	Oral	10−20 ml twice daily	52
Magnesium sulphate (Epsom salts)		Oral	5−10 g/day	52

Generic name	Proprietary name	Route of administration	Dose range	Page no.
Constipation cont'd				
Stimulant laxatives				
Bisacodyl	Dulcolax	Oral	10−20 mg/day	52
Cascara		Oral	1−3 tabs/day	52
Danthron	Co-danthrusate (danthron+docusate)	Oral	1−3 caps/day	52
Docusate	Dioctyl	Oral	100−500 mg/day	52
Senna		Oral	2−4 tabs/day	52
Sodium picosulphate	Picolax	Oral	5−15 ml/day	52
Convulsions				60,124
Carbamazepine	Tegretol	Oral	0.1−1.2 g/day	60
Dexamethasone	Decadron	Oral/s.c.	2−16 mg/day	60
Diazepam	Diazemuls	i.v.	10−20 mg	60
	Stesolid	p.r.	10−20 mg	60
Phenobarbitone	Luminal	Oral	30−180 mg/day	60
Phenytoin	Epanutin	Oral	100−600 mg/day	60
Sodium valproate	Epilim	Oral	0.6−2.5 g/day	60
Cough				58
Acetylcysteine	Fabrol	Oral	200 mg thrice daily	58
Carbocisteine	Mucodyne	Oral	0.75−1.5 g/day	58
Codeine linctus		Oral	5−10 ml thrice daily	58
Diamorphine linctus		Oral	2.5−10 ml 4-hourly	58
Methadone linctus		Oral	2.5−5 ml 4-hourly	58
Salbutamol	Ventolin	Oral	2−4 mg four times daily	58
		Inhaled	2 puffs four times daily	
		Nebulised	2.5 mg four times daily	
Depression				68−72
Amitriptyline	Tryptizol	Oral	50−200 mg/day	71
Butriptyline	Evadyne	Oral	75−150 mg/day	71
Clomipramine	Anafranil	Oral	30−150 mg/day	70,71
Desipramine	Pertofran	Oral	75−200 mg/day	70,71
Dexamphetamine	Dexedrine	Oral	5−15 mg/day	71,72
Dothiepin	Prothiaden	Oral	75−150 mg/day	71
Doxepin	Sinequan	Oral	75−300 mg/day	71
Imipramine	Tofranil	Oral	75−200 mg/day	70,71
Iprindole	Prondol	Oral	15−60 mg thrice daily	71
Isocarboxazid	Marplan	Oral	10−30 mg/day	71
Maprotiline	Ludiomil	Oral	25−150 mg/day	71
Mianserin	Bolvidon	Oral	30−200 mg/day	71
Nortriptyline	Aventyl	Oral	20−100 mg/day	71
Phenelzine	Nardil	Oral	30−60 mg/day	71
Protriptyline	Concordin	Oral	15−60 mg/day	71
Tranylcypromine	Parnate	Oral	10−30 mg/day	71
Trimipramine	Surmontil	Oral	50−300 mg/day	71

Generic name	Proprietary name	Route of administration	Dose range	Page no.
Diarrhoea				53,103
Codeine phosphate		Oral	10 – 300 mg/day	53
Diphenoxylate	Lomotil	Oral	10 mg then 5 mg 4-hourly	53
Ispaghula	Fybogel	Oral	1 – 4 sachet/day	53
Kaolin				
Loperamide	Imodium	Oral	6 – 16 mg/day	53
Methylcellulose	Celevac	Oral	3 – 6 tabs/day	53
Sterculia	Normacol	Oral	1 – 4 sachet/day	53
Dysphagia				56 – 57,102
Dexamethasone	Decadron	Oral/s.c.	2 – 16 mg/day	56
Ketoconazole	Nizoral	Oral	200 – 400 mg daily	56
Dyspnoea				58 – 59,102
Diazepam	Valium	Oral	2 – 5 mg thrice daily	58
Morphine		Oral/s.c.	2.5 – 5 mg 4-hourly	58
Haemoptysis				59,124
Diamorphine			Related to previous dose	124
Diazepam	Diazemuls	i.v.	10 – 20 mg	124
Hiccup				56
Chlorpromazine	Largactil	i.v.	25 mg + 25 mg i.m.	56
Metoclopramide	Maxolon	Oral	10 mg thrice daily	56
Hypercalcaemia				51,56 – 66, 124
Dexamethasone	Decadron	Oral/s.c.	2 – 16 mg/day	66
Frusemide	Lasix	Oral	40 mg/day	66
Mithramycin	Mithracin	Oral	25 μg/kg	66,124
Sodium cellulose phosphate	Calcisorb	Oral	5 g thrice daily	66
Insomnia				59 – 60
Alcohol				59
Nitrazepam	Mogadon	Oral	5 – 10 mg at night	60
Temazepam	Normison	Oral	10 – 30 mg at night	60
Triazolam	Halcion	Oral	250 μg at night	
Intestinal obstruction				51 – 55
Cyclizine	Valoid	Oral	50 mg twice or thrice daily	51,55
Dexamethasone	Decadron	Oral/s.c.	2 – 16 mg/day	55
Docusate	Dioctyl	Oral	100 – 500 mg/day	55
Haloperidol	Haldol	Oral	5 – 10 mg/day	55
Hyoscine		Oral/s.c.	400 μg thrice daily	51,55
Methotrimeprazine	Nozinan	s.c.	25 – 200 mg/day	55
Propantheline	Pro-Banthine	Oral	15 mg thrice daily	55

Generic name	Proprietary name	Route of administration	Dose range	Page no.
Mouth problems				42,54,103
Amphotericin	Fungilin	Oral	100−200 mg four times daily	54,103
Hydrocortisone	Corlan	Oral	2.5 mg lozenges four times daily	54
Ketoconazole	Nizoral	Oral	200−400 mg daily	54,103
Metoclopramide	Maxolon	Oral	10 mg thrice daily	54
Metronidazole	Flagyl	Oral	0.2−1 g thrice daily	54
Nystatin	Nystan	Oral	up to 0.5 units four times daily	54
Nausea and vomiting				36,49−51
Chlorpromazine	Largactil	Oral/i.m. p.r.	25−50 mg thrice daily 100 mg thrice daily	
Cinnarizine	Stugeron	Oral	30 mg thrice daily	50
Cyclizine	Valoid	Oral	50 mg twice or thrice daily	50,51
Dexamethasone	Decadron	Oral/s.c.	2−16 mg/day	50,51
Domperidone	Motilium	Oral	10−40 mg thrice daily	50,51
Fluphenazine	Moditen	Oral	1−2 mg twice daily	51
Haloperidol	Haldol	Oral	5−10 mg/day	50,51
Hyoscine		Oral/s.c.	400 μg thrice daily	50
Methotrimeprazine	Nozinan	s.c.	25−200 mg/day	50
Metoclopramide	Maxolon	Oral i.v./s.c.	10 mg thrice daily up to 10 mg/kg/day	50 50,51
Nabilone	Cesamet	Oral	1 mg twice daily	50
Prochlorperazine	Stemetil	Oral	5 mg thrice daily	51
Pain				4,36, 42−48
Amitriptyline	Tryptizol	Oral	25−75 mg twice daily	46
Aspirin		Oral	300−900 mg 4-hourly	45,46
Buprenorphine	Temgesic	s/l	200−400 μg 3−4 times daily	46
Carbamazepine	Tegretol	Oral	100−200 mg thrice daily	46
Codeine		Oral	30−60 mg 4-hourly	45
Dexamethasone	Decadron	Oral/s.c.	2−16 mg/day	46
Dextromoramide	Palfium	Oral/s.c./p.r.	5−20 mg for acute episodes of pain	46
Dextropropoxyphene	Co-Proxamol	Oral	2 tabs four times daily	45,46
Diamorphine		Oral/s.c.	2.5−q.s. 4-hourly	45,46,47
Diazepam	Valium	Oral/i.v./p.r.	2−10 mg 3−4 times daily	46
Morphine		Oral/s.c.	2.5−q.s. 4-hourly	45,46,47
NSAIDs	Brufen	Oral	1.2−1.8 g/day	45,46
	Indocid	Oral/ p.r.	50−200 mg/day 100 mg at night	
	Naprosyn	Oral p.r.	0.5−1 g/day 500 mg at night	
Paracetamol		Oral	0.5−1 g 4-hourly	45
Sodium valproate	Epilim	Oral	0.6−2.5 g/day	46

Generic name	Proprietary name	Route of administration	Dose range	Page no.
Pruritus				63
Cholestyramine	Qestran	Oral	4–8 g/day	63
Dexamethasone	Decadron	Oral/s.c.	2–16 mg/day	63
Haloperidol	Haldol	Oral	0.5 mg thrice daily or 2 mg at night	63
Methyltestosterone		Oral	10 mg thrice daily	63
Stanozolol	Stromba	Oral	5 mg/day	63
Skin lesions				46,63,104
Hydrogen peroxide				63
KY gel				63
Metronidazole				46,63
Povidone-iodine				46,63
Squashed stomach syndrome				57
Aluminium hydroxide	Asilone	Oral	2 tab thrice daily	57
Metoclopramide	Maxolon	Oral	10 mg thrice daily	57
Sweating (excessive)				63
Cimetidine	Tagamet	Oral	200 mg thrice daily	63
Indomethacin	Indocid	Oral	25 mg thrice daily	63
Paracetamol		Oral	0.5–1 g 4-hourly	63
Propranolol	Inderal	Oral	10–40 mg thrice daily	63
Taste problems				55
Zinc	Zincomed	Oral	220 mg thrice daily	55

NB Zinc deficient individuals cannot distinguish between a 0.1% $ZnSO_4$ solution and water

Generic name	Proprietary name	Route of administration	Dose range	Page no.
Tenesmus				54
Chlorpromazine	Largactil	Oral	25–50 mg thrice daily	54
Terminal respiratory symptoms				123–124
Diamorphine		s.c.	Depending on previous dosage	124
Hyoscine		s.c.	400 μg	124
Urinary symptoms				64–65
Amitriptyline	Tryptizol	Oral	25–75 mg twice daily	64
Chlorhexidine		Bladder washout		64
Flavoxate	Urispas	Oral	200 mg thrice daily	64
Propantheline	Pro-Banthine	Oral	15–30 mg thrice daily	64
Terodiline	Terolin	Oral	12.5–25 mg twice daily	61
Vertigo				61
Cinnarizine	Stugeron	Oral	30 mg thrice daily	61
Cyclizine	Valoid	Oral	50 mg twice or thrice daily	61
Hyoscine		Oral/s.c.	400 μg thrice daily	61
Metoclopramide	Maxolon	Oral	10 mg thrice daily	61

i.m. = intramuscularly; i.v. = intravenously; p.r. = per rectum; q.s. = quid sufficient (enough); s.c. = subcutaneously; s.l. = sublingually.

Appendix 2: Addresses of helping organizations

Age Concern
Bernard Sunley House
60 Pitcairn Road
Mitcham
Surrey CR4 3LL
Tel. 01 640 5431

Local branches may be able to offer bereavement counselling. Also publish free fact sheet on arranging a funeral. Have combined with CRUSE to publish *Survival Guide for Widows* (£3.50 + p.p.).

AIDS Helpline
Tel. 0800 567 123

Offers information and advice to any caller on all aspects of AIDS. A 24-hour, free, confidential serivce.

Association of Carers
Medway Homes
Belfour Road
Rochester
Kent

A national association offering support to carers of relatives with any disability or illness through advice, counselling, welfare rights information and a network of local groups. They publish *Help at Hand*, a signpost guide to benefits and services for carers.

BACUP
121/3 Charterhouse Street
London EC1 M6AA

British Association of Cancer United Patients provides information, advice and support to cancer patients and their families and friends.

Benevolent Societies
Soldiers, Sailors and
   Airmen's Family
   Association (SSAFA)
16−18 Old Queen Street
London SW1H 9HP

For patients who have served in the Forces and who may need some help. Financial assistance may be available.

Earl Haig Fund
48 Pall Mall
London SW1Y 5JY

RAF Benevolent Fund
67 Portland Place
London W1N 4AR

**Breastcare and
  Mastectomy Association**
26A Harrison Street
(off Grays Inn Road)
Kings Cross
London WC1H 8JG
Tel. 01 837 0908

Concerned with all aspects of breast
cancer. Offers a non-medical service
staffed by experienced volunteers.

**British Colostomy
  Association**
4th Floor
38 Eccleston Square
London SW1V 1PB
Tel. 01 828 5175

Produces a range of information leaflets as
well as volunteers who will talk to people
with newly diagnosed bowel cancer.

British Red Cross Society
see local telephone directory

May be able to help with loans of
equipment such as wheelchairs, commodes,
walking aids, etc. Some branches also
provide 'house-bound clubs' and holidays
for disable people (not just cancer
patients). Local branches nationwide.

Cancer Link
46 Pentonville Road
London N1 9HF

Provides information and emotional
support for people with cancer and their
relatives and friends. Also publishes
directories of useful organizations and
cancer support groups.

**Cancer Relief
  Macmillan Fund**
Anchor House
15/19 Britten Street
London SW3 3TY

National charity for cancer sufferers and
their families. Can provide financial
assistance. Also establishes and funds a
number of Macmillan Home Care Services
throughout Britain. Application may be
made by health visitors, community
nurses, Macmillan nurses or social
workers for assistance with such things as
fuel bills, special foods or bus fares.

CHAT
20 Cavendish Square
London W1M 0AB
Tel. 01 629 3870

Counselling, Help and Advice Together
provide an independent, confidential
counselling service based at the Royal
College of Nursing.

Compassionate Friends
6 Denmark Street
Bristol BS1 5DQ
Tel. 0272 292 778

Nationwide organization of parents who have had a child die. Offers friendship and understanding to other bereaved parents.

CRUSE
Cruse House
126 Sheen Road
Richmond
Surrey TW9 1UR

A national charity which was founded to help people who are bereaved. Local groups exist in most towns. These offer skilled counsellors, social workers, group meetings, social groups. They may be contacted prior to the bereavement if necessary.

Disabled Living Foundation
380/384 Harrow Road
London W9 2HO
Tel. 01 289 6111

Advice on equipment for disabled.

Hospices

Information about hospices can be provided by the general practitioner or hospital consultant who normally refer the patient.

Hospice Information Service
51/53 Lawrie Park Road
Sydenham SE26 6DZ

Can provide further information about location of nearest hospice and the facilities provided. Can also supply bibliographies and additional reading material upon request to the librarian.

Ileostomy Association of GB and Ireland
Amblehurst House
Black Scotch Lane
Mansfield
Nottinghamshire NG18 4PF

Support groups throughout the country. Also publishes quarterly journal.

Let's Face It
PO Box 400
London W3 5XJ

Provides a support network for people with facial handicap.

London Lighthouse
111/117 Lancaster Road
London W11 1QT
Tel. 01 792 1200

AIDS hospice.

**Malcolm Sargent Cancer
Fund**
6 Sydney Street
London SW3 6PP

Provides financial assistance to help
children suffering from cancer, leukaemia
and Hodgkin's disease.

Marie Curie Foundation
124 Sloane Street
London SW1 9BP
or
21 Rutland Street
Edinburgh EH1 2AE

A national cancer charity which provides
nursing homes to provide pain and
symptom control. Also can provide respite
care and accommodation for patients
attending radiotherapy centres. The
Foundation can also fund nurses to care
for patients in their own homes,
particularly at night.

Motor Neurone Disease
38 Hazelwood Road
Northamptom NN1 1LN

Can offer financial advice and practical
support for motor neurone disease
patients. They will give details of local
groups and publish leaflets to help
relatives.

**National Association of
Laryngectomy Clubs**
4th Floor
39 Eccleston Square
London SW1V 1PB
Tel. 01 834 2857

Association of 51 clubs; offers help and
advice directly to patients before and after
their operations. Also produces a card for
laryngectomees to carry, outlining the
ncessary procedure for resuscitation in an
emergency.

Nurses Support Group
Tel. 01 708 5605
(Mon/Wed
7.00 p.m. – 10.00 p.m.)

Provides help and advice to HIV + nurses.

Samaritans
See local telephone
directory

Provides a confidential listening service.

Seekers Trust
The Close
Addington Park
Maidstone
Kent ME19 5BL
Tel. 0732 843 589

A community for healing through prayer.

SPOD
286 Camden Road
London N7 0BJ
Tel. 01 607 8851/2

Provides advice, counselling and useful leaflets on sexual problems for anyone with a disability, not just cancer.

Tenovus Cancer
Information Centre
11 Whitchurch Road
Cardiff CF3 3JN

Produce a number of booklets about cancer in general, such as *Cancer Answers* and *Hopeful Facts about Cancer*.

Terrence Higgins Trust
52 – 54 Grays Inn Road
London WC1X 8JU
Tel. 01 831 0330

Provides information on AIDS and help and advice to sufferers and anyone worried about the disease.
Helpline 01 833 2971
(7.00 p.m. – 10.00 p.m. weekdays;
 3.00 p.m. – 10.00 p.m. weekends)

Urostomy Association
Buckland
Beaumont Park
Danbury
Essex CM3 4DE
Tel. 024 541 4294

Publishes journal in the spring and autumn

Appendix 3: The question of euthanasia

In March 1988, following the publication of a Mori poll whose findings are summarized in Table A.1, one of us (RH) attended a press meeting with members of both houses at the House of Commons. The statement made to that meeting represents our views on euthanasia, but it is recognized and respected that others hold different views. The debate about euthanasia is likely to become very important at the end of this century as demographic changes in the population and increased life expectancy of cancer patients swell the numbers of patients needing palliative care.

Statement to the House of Commons Press Conference, March 1988

After 25 years as a general practitioner in Warwickshire I spent three years as Professor of General Practice in a University in Amsterdam and I am currently working in the hospice movement. This has given me experience of patients undergoing protracted death from chronic conditions such as cancer and has exposed me to many occasions when doctors, patients, their relatives or sometimes I myself have raised the question of euthanasia. The word, of course, means 'good death' and as such is something we must all wish for. However, euthanasia has come to mean 'assisted death' which is simply a euphemism for homicide.

I can understand the views of those who argue for the legalization of such assisted death, indeed I even subscribed to them myself at an earlier stage in my career, but now I believe those views to be wrong. That does not mean I doubt the sincerity of those who hold them.

It is an unusual state of affairs for a patient to request death. Perhaps the most common reason is depression then, because of an acute illness the patient's view of him (or herself) is distorted. In such an abnormal state the patient regards himself as worthless, perhaps even a burden to his immediate family and sees his death as the best solution to an apparently intolerable situation. Such a state of affairs is a common manifestation of mental illness and one which is presented to family doctors frequently.

Faced with such a case the doctor could do nothing, in which case most patients will slowly recover but a significant proportion would commit suicide. The doctor, realizing the patient's agony of mind could give him a prescription for a lethal quantity of tablets, or even a revolver with a single round of ammunition. A third option is open to the doctor; he might by using all his skills of communication, empathy and care, by mobilizing all the supportive resources within the patient's family and environment and by the judicious use of drugs, intervene in the illness and alter the patient's view of himself, his worth and the usefulness of his life. If the doctor is successful in the attempt the wish for death will pass and, as the patient recovers, the threat of violence against himself will disappear.

This may sound very obvious, you may feel that no doctor would ever give his patient a loaded gun; perhaps not, but many provide an equally lethal prescription and in Amsterdam I have heard it argued that putting the means of suicide into a patient's hands is justifiable if that is what the patient really wants. This is carrying respect for the patient's autonomy to extremes. I argue that in such a case the death wish is the product of the illness and that the doctor's job is to remove the pathological reason for wanting death rather than to acquiesce with the patient's intention.

Ah, you will say, that is quite different from a no hope situation, depression is treatable, or may get better by itself, cancer and a number of other diseases are not like that. For where one is faced by the inevitability of death, is it not better to die sooner rather than bear an agony of pain? This question is the crux of the Mori poll of 1808 individuals recorded by December 1987 to which it produced a generally affirmative answer. The trouble with this poll is that it questioned within the framework of popular and uninformed belief. Unfortunately cancer is surrounded by a dense cloak · of superstition and myth; the questions in the Mori poll were asked of people who do not work regularly with cancer and who neither understand the nature of pain nor how it can be relieved.

'Pain' is a very inadequate word. We all think we know what it means yet since we all have such varied experience of pain we probably all mean something different by the word. The pain of advanced cancer is different in every case so that a single word is useless to convey its range of meaning. Perhaps 'anguish' is better to describe the complex mixture of physical, psychological, social and spiritual distress which occurs in cancer patients. To many it comes as a surprise that properly researched studies indicate that a third of all cancer patients do not suffer physical pain (and non-cancerous terminal disease is even more frequently pain-free) but all suffer the emotional anguish; fear, anger, grief, or guilt, they may also be distressed at their loss of independence and autonomy, they may be desperately bored at their enforced inactivity, they may have financial or relationship worries and will be undergoing bereavement at the inevitability of separation from loved ones. Add to this spiritual doubt and religious confusion that the God in whom they trusted has apparently deserted them, and the true meaning of anguish becomes apparent.

But there is an enormous amount that can be done by the careful analysis of each and every component of the individual's anguish. I have seen many people change with a skilful management from the indignity of an overwhelming anguish to a state of comfort, even of happiness—that is the true meaning of euthanasia, good death. That this can be achieved in the vast majority of cases has been clearly demonstrated by the work of hospices but it has to be said that such attention to detail is costly in time, in manpower and in money. Still only a small proportion of cancer patients receive the benefit of such care during their last weeks.

Of course euthanasia is easy and cheap. My profession has been rightly criticized for the way in which it used tranquillizer drugs in the past; it was always easier and cheaper to write a prescription for Valium than to listen to the patients and try to sort out their muddled lives, a process which may consume many hours. The proper care of the terminally sick is even more time-consuming, and how attractively expediency beckons so that killing may become the tranquillizer of terminal illness. That is the beginning of a slippery slope which, in an ever aging society, leads to a final solution for the old, the infirm or the mentally defective.

Alteration of the law is not the answer, indeed it will only create problems. What is needed is education of the public with regard to cancer and other terminal diseases and about what can be done for those who suffer from them.

Education is also badly needed by the medical profession into improved methods of the care of patients with advanced disease, especially cancer. The hospices are too few to deal with all the workload but they must assume responsibility for leading the thrust of medical education so that 'good death' bcomes an integral part of both good general and specialist practice.

That way there will seldom if ever be the need for assisted death.

Robin Hull   23.3.88

Appendix 4: Mori poll: opinions on euthanasia

Mori poll: opinions on euthanasia (Based on a sample of 1808 individuals in December 1987).

1 In how many cases would you say that a person who is terminally ill could be almost totally free of pain through the use of drugs?

In:

All cases	9%
Most cases	41%
About half the cases	14%
A few cases	20%
No cases	4%
Don't know	14%

2 In Holland, some doctors carry out euthanasia when their patients request it, by giving sedatives and injecting muscle relaxants so as to paralyse breathing. Some people have said the law in Britain should be changed so as to allow euthanasia in some circumstances, as is done in Holland. Others believe the law should not be changed. Which of the following options comes closest to your view.

(a) Euthanasia should be made legal in all cases when the patient requests it	23%
(b) Euthanasia should be made legal only when a patient who requests it is suffering from a severe illness and is in a lot of pain	49%
(c) The law should not be changed so as to allow euthanasia	19%
(d) Don't know	9%

3 If euthanasia were practised in Britain more people would be frightened to go to hospital.

Agree	44%
Neutral	8%
Disagree	42%
Don't know	6%

4 Because it is currently illegal for doctors in Britain to terminate the lives of their patients, patients need never fear that they will do so.

Agree	62%
Neutral	12%
Disagree	15%
Don't know	11%

5 If euthanasia was available on request to patients who are permanently dependent on others for medical or nursing care, some would choose it so as not to be a burden on others.

Agree	71%
Neutral	6%
Disagree	12%
Don't know	10%

6 In cases where a patient is unable to communicate with others, it should be legal for the patient's next of kin to request euthanasia on their behalf.

Agree	31%
Neutral	11%
Disagree	47%
Don't know	11%

7 If a patient requests euthanasia a doctor should always be obliged to carry it out.

Agree	40%
Neutral	11%
Disagree	41%
Don't know	9%

Conclusion

Though two-thirds of the public regard terminal illness as being rendered relatively painless through the use of drugs in at least half the terminal illness cases, a significant majority are nevertheless in favour of legalizing euthanasia—particularly in cases where illness and pain are severe. However, the obligation of doctors to carry out patient-request euthanasia as part of their contract is by no means universally acceptable to the public.

There is some concern among the public, and particularly concern for elderly people, that if euthanasia was practised in Britain people would be frightened to go into hospital. There is considerable opposition to patients' next of kin being allowed to make decisions regarding euthanasia for the patient.

Further reading

Worcester, R.M., Corrado, M. & Allen, R. (1988) *Public Attitudes to Euthanasia*. Market & Opinion Research International Ltd, London.

Index

Drugs are *not* included in this index but will be found listed by indication in Appendix 1.